INT.

Welcome to the So Connected® Mental Strength Coaching Journal For Athletes Book 2.

In Book 1 of So Connected® Mental Strength Coaching Journal For Athletes we practiced connecting our mind to our body. In this book, we will focus on connecting our own inner resources to our goals. We want to take our mental strength into our future by achieving every goal we set out to accomplish.

You'll learn how to wrap your head around your talent and share it with the world!

Being more of *you* in *your* life is a practice.

I cannot wait to see what you accomplish when you tap into your potential and OWN IT.

— Stacey

Copyright © 2020 by Stacey Herman Goodrich
All rights reserved. This book or any portion thereof
may not be reproduced or used in any manner
without the express written permission of the author
except for the use of brief quotations in a book review.

ISBN: 978-1-7354571-1-6

Printed in the United States of America

Designed by Kirstie Walheim

JOIN THE GROUP

Please join my Facebook group:
Mental Strength Coaching Journal For Athletes

It's for you, the person using this journal. Ask me questions, talk with others on the same journey, and surround yourself with support.

Additional Facebook group support:
Athletes Who Settle For More

Social Media:
www.so-connected.com
@ stacey_connected
@ConnectedStacey
Athletes Who Settle For More

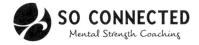

This book belongs to

_____

As I put more of me into my A Circle, and communicate from that perspective, I am more whole and I can achieve anything I put my mind to.

TABLE OF
Contents

3 — INTRODUCTION

5 — JOIN THE GROUP

9 — SNAPSHOT OF THE PROCESS

11 — THE PROCESS

11 — STEP 1: CHOOSE YOUR INTENTIONAL
          WORD OF THE DAY

14 — STEP 2: THE STRATEGIES –
          PRACTICING YOUR SUCCESS

15 — THE DOING STRATEGY®

17 — THE LEARNING STRATEGY®

18 — A-CIRCLE STRATEGY®

22 — STEP 3: GOALS IN MOTION

22 — GOAL BEYOND THE GOAL®

24 — STEP 4: STRATEGIES FOR SUCCESS

28 — STEP 5: PURGE IT. VENT. GET IT OUT!

30 — 1ST MONTH JOURNALING SECTION

102 — 2ND MONTH JOURNALING SECTION

174 — 3RD MONTH JOURNALING SECTION

247 — STICKER PAGE

BRINGING CONSCIOUS AWARENESS TO YOUR

UNCONSCIOUS
RECIPE FOR SUCCESS

EQUALS

WRAPPING YOUR HEAD AROUND YOUR TALENT.

LIVE IN YOUR POTENTIAL!

© Stacey Herman Goodrich

SNAPSHOT OF THE PROCESS

1 **INTENTIONAL WORD OF THE DAY**
Work your mindset daily! Pick a word or phrase that you connect with. Use the intentional word of the day to reset your mentality. It keeps you intentional in the moment and gives you the choice to be in charge. Focus on where you want to be!

2 **THE STRATEGIES –PRACTICING YOUR SUCCESS**
Doing Strategy®, **Learning** Strategy®, and **A-Circle**® **O**!
Strategies give you the *how* —how to duplicate success and perform in your potential over time.

3 **GOALS IN MOTION**
Small daily goals align your mind and body. A **Goal Beyond The Goal**® will give you purpose (the why) of your day-to-day responsibilities. Over time your results show your success.

4 **STRATEGIES FOR SUCCESS**
What do you do well and how do you do it well? Connecting your unconscious strategy for success to your behavior, using this strategy to align with your goals (and your goal beyond the goal), is the process you need to perform in your potential. Tap into your talent one day at a time.

5 **PURGE IT ALL! GET IT OUT!**
Purge it all! Get it out! As you do –replace it with what you want now! Let's dig in!

GIVE YOURSELF PERMISSION TO NOT BE PERFECT SO YOU CAN BECOME MORE EXCELLENT!

© Stacey Herman Goodrich

THE PROCESS

STEP 1 CHOOSE YOUR INTENTIONAL WORD OF THE DAY

Pick a word or phrase that connects to you... each day. Pick one listed on the next page or one of your own! The ability to control your mindset, in the moment, is important. We can all be affected by our situations; this strategy keeps us focused.

Here is an example of how to use the Intentional Word Of The Day. Let's use the phrase, "fresh start." Imagine you are a player on a softball team, and a teammate has an at-bat that isn't positive, you could say, "fresh start!"

This resets your teammate's mentality. It stops the negative thoughts and actions, and allows them to choose to change it! It's a way to practice adjusting perspective in the moment. Does that make sense? Resetting your mentality with an intentional word of the day puts you in charge. It gives you power over the moment.

Your present situation may be stressful or chaotic, but choosing to shift your thoughts to your goals can help. Think of it as separating your "present self" from your "goal self." In the moment, you can decide to focus on what you need to do to move toward your goals instead of being caught up in the annoyance of your situation. The Intentional Word Of The Day can keep you connected to your goals, even in a moment of distress.

Practicing this strategy on a day-to-day basis allows us to be in charge of our situation, choose our behaviors and thoughts, and can help us be more successful over time. This journal gives you the ability to acknowledge it, track it, and get better at it!

SUGGESTIONS FOR THE WORD OF THE DAY

Below are words that you can use, but feel free to use whatever word works for you on a day-to-day basis.

When you affirm words it is helpful, but intentionally connecting words to your behavior is EMPOWERING YOUR POWER!

I suggest you do this personally and add it to your team to bring more success.

WORD SUGGESTIONS

Connected	Faith	Commitment
Movement	Fearless	Mindset
Goal	Drive	Motivation
Knowledgeable	Abundance	Accomplish
Accountability	Graceful	Refined
Choice	Meaningful	Fresh Start
Express	Happy	Open-minded
Belief	Opportunity	Creative
Captivate	Healthy	Positivity
Optimism	Thankful	Strength
Legacy	Illuminate	Harmony
Support	Attitude	Thoughtful
Determination	Joy	Grateful
Genuine	Intention	Wisdom
Love	Excellent	Leadership
Essence	Kindness	Mentally Strong
Openhearted	Eager	Acceptance
Extraordinary	Legendary	Grit
Togetherness	Fabulous	Strategies

WHEN YOU AFFIRM WORDS IT IS HELPFUL, BUT INTENTIONALLY CONNECTING WORDS TO YOUR BEHAVIOR IS *EMPOWERING* *YOUR POWER*

© Stacey Herman Goodrich

STEP 2 THE STRATEGIES – PRACTICING YOUR SUCCESS

Everybody has strategies. Strategies are used to be successful or unsuccessful, to get what we want, or what we don't want. A common problem is that most people are unaware of the strategy they are using, therefore, they cannot control their outcomes consistently. Strategies are happening at the unconscious level or automatically.

Is it frustrating for you when you know what to do to be successful, but it doesn't turn out the way you want? Have you practiced the skill/play/game enough to provide success, but the result is still lacking?

The **Doing Strategy®**, the **Learning Strategy®**, and **A-Circle®** are strategies that will give you options to manage situations better. Learning and understanding these strategies will help you get the results you want.

IF JUST TELLING YOU TO BE CONFIDENT, NOT TO WORRY ABOUT IT, TO GET OUT OF YOUR HEAD, WORKED — WE WOULD ALL BE PERFECT.

© Stacey Herman Goodrich

DOING STRATEGY®

THE DOING STRATEGY® IS WHEN YOUR MIND IS NOT IN YOUR WAY, YOUR BODY KNOWS WHAT TO DO, AND YOU CAN JUST DO IT.

When you first started practicing your sport, you didn't have to think about what you were doing, you just did it! You picked up a ball and threw it (maybe not accurately), you did a cartwheel (maybe not perfectly), you jumped in the pool to swim (maybe not gracefully).

Most people "do" their skills/plays/game for many years but it's happening automatically, so consciously they are unable to use its potential. At this point, because it is an unconscious strategy, when something goes wrong, they don't know what to do or how to fix it.

I had a client who played football, and he said to me, "I can kick a football straight through the upright over and over again in practice, but when I get to a game, or a pressure situation, I can't do it." His coaches would keep saying, "Don't worry about it, just get out of your head."

If telling people, "don't worry about it, just get out of your head" or "just be confident you can do it" worked, we would all be perfectly consistent, right?

For my client, the football athlete (I will call him Joe), when he was practicing, he was basically just doing it. He just kicked the ball and didn't really have to think about it. Then in a game, or pressure situation, just doing it didn't work. When this happened Joe did not know what to do. Typically when just "doing it" doesn't work for people, it is common for them to mentally bail out and get stuck.

I told Joe, "If you can just do your skills/game (kicks) **without a lot of thought**, that is an option. That is the Doing Strategy®."

Bringing awareness to what was working for him in the past ("doing" his kick), giving it a name (the Doing Strategy®), allows him to consider it (I have an option), practice it (I am going to just do my skill without a lot of thought), and maximize its potential (owning it!)

Understanding the Doing Strategy® provides a mental connection to what to do physically *in the moment.* This is an option, and a solution.

Where in the past did you just do your skills/plays/game? Can you now see where you could have used the Doing Strategy®? Can you see how when moving forward you can just do your skills without much thought? In this journal, you will be able to practice this idea to support yourself.

Typically, with athletes, there is a situation where just "doing it" doesn't work. It could be when you are on a new/better team and you're worried about what the coach is thinking, or you have a high expectation of yourself and that idea gets in your way, preventing you from doing what you want. For Joe, it was the pressure situation where just "doing it" did not work. He needed another option. I taught him the Learning Strategy®.

DOING STRATEGY®
IS JUST DOING IT WITHOUT
A LOT OF THOUGHT.
© Stacey Herman Goodrich

LEARNING STRATEGY®
KEEPS YOUR MIND
CONNECTED TO YOUR BODY.
© Stacey Herman Goodrich

LEARNING STRATEGY®

THE LEARNING STRATEGY® IS FOCUSING ON YOUR SKILL/PLAY/GAME ONE PIECE AT A TIME OR HOW YOU ARE DOING IT IN THE MOMENT.

The Learning Strategy® is focusing on your skill/play/game one piece at a time, or how you are doing it in the moment. It is not thinking about what you *need* to do, and then trying to do it. It is thinking about what you *want* to do, *as you are doing it.*

When I taught this strategy to Joe, I said, "Joe, when you are kicking the ball in practice, what are you thinking about?" He said, "Nothing, I am just doing it." I said, "Okay, when you are kicking the ball in practice, what do you want to be focusing on so that when you kick in the game, you are mentally prepared?" He said, "I want to focus on how I connect my foot to the ball, my technique, and my follow-through." I said, "Great. Can you practice it that way so when you are in a game you are mentally ready?" He said, "Yes."

The Learning Strategy® is focusing on your technique, form, or mechanics. It is thinking about HOW you want to do it physically. It keeps your mind connected to your body, supporting what you are doing, AS YOU ARE DOING IT.

Do you ever feel like your mind and your body are not on the same page? Do you ever have negative thoughts controlling you?

When things don't go right, negative thoughts can get in our way. If we do not give our mind a job to do, it can create its own job, and sometimes it might not be helpful. Sometimes our mind might be thinking about what we don't want to happen, what we are worried about, or what our coaches are thinking. Unfortunately, this disconnects our mind from our body, causing us issues physically.

The Learning Strategy® gives your mind a job to focus on, **what you want,** instead of what you do not want to happen. It's a strategy that connects your mind to your body.

Think back to situations that did not go well for you. Do you see how using the Learning Strategy® could have been helpful, — a way you could have approached it one step at a time? In this journal we will explore this, and work with it, to help you create more success.

A-CIRCLE STRATEGY®

A-CIRCLE® PROVIDES US THE CAPABILITY TO BE AWARE OF WHAT IS CONTROLLING US, AND GIVES US THE ABILITY TO MANAGE IT.

Many times we have situations where what is controlling us is not what we want. Sometimes negative thoughts, limiting beliefs, and anxiety/pressure/stress can be running the show. It is difficult because obviously we don't want this, but again it is happening unconsciously. Have you ever had a coach tell you, "get out of your head," or "you are over-thinking it"? Just because the coach did not have a solution for you, doesn't mean there isn't one. **There is nothing wrong with your mind and you are not the problem.** A-Circle® provides us the capability to be aware of what is controlling us, and gives us the ability to manage it.

Everyone has a mental A Circle, B Circle, and C Circle. (See diagram on page 19)

A Circle: Whoever or whatever is in your A Circle is who or what is making decisions for you, or who or what is running the show for you in that particular situation.

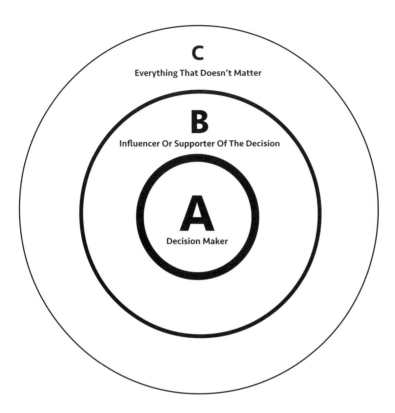

Diagram of A-CIRCLE STRATEGY®
© Stacey Herman Goodrich

A CIRCLE	**B** CIRCLE	**C** CIRCLE
Who or what is making decisions for you, or who or what is running the show for you in that particular situation.	People or things that influence your decisions, or they can support you to make a decision, but they're not actually making it for you.	Everyone and everything outside of your A and B Circle, or everything that doesn't matter or is irrelevant.

B Circle: Contains people or things that influence your decisions, or they can support you to make a decision, but they're not actually making it for you.

C Circle: Contains everyone and everything outside of your A and B Circle, or everything that doesn't matter or is irrelevant.

We can have lots of things in our A Circle —we can have people, thoughts, and/or energy. You may have your coaches, family, and/or teammates in your A Circle in certain situations. You may or may not be in your own A Circle at times. Do you worry about making a mistake, or what people think of you? These ideas could be in your A Circle and controlling you at times, correct? Do you play well in practice, but in a game, pressure jumps into your A Circle? — similar to Joe's situation. Have you experienced a time when worry, anxiety, or injury were in your A Circle? Do you see how in those situations it was controlling you?

We can also manage what we want in our A Circle. We can kick everything out, and just do our skills (the Doing Strategy®), we can focus on one thing at a time (the Learning Strategy®), we can have confidence, people who support us, and belief in ourselves, in our A Circle.

The same day that I taught Joe the Doing Strategy® and the Learning Strategy®, I taught him A-Circle®. I said to him, "Joe, everybody has an A Circle, B Circle, and C Circle. There is no right or wrong way with how it is set up. It is a way for us to understand what's running the show in any given situation. Whoever or whatever is in your A Circle is who or what is making decisions for you. Your B Circle contains people or things that influence your decisions, or they can support you to make a decision, but they're not making it for you.
C Circle contains everything else outside of that —everything else irrelevant."

I asked Joe, "When you think back to the game where you couldn't kick the ball correctly, what was in your A Circle?" He said, "I was worried that I was going to mess up." I said to him, "Do you see how that idea was controlling you?" He said, "Yes." I said, "In that situation, what could you have had in your A Circle?" He said, "I could have just been focusing on how I needed to kick the ball." I said, "Do you see how that would have been different for you?" He said, "Yes."

Think back to a situation in your sport that didn't go well. Who or what was in your A Circle? What could you have had in your A Circle back then? Moving forward, what do you want to have in your A Circle?

These are some of the questions we will process throughout this journal. Do not worry if you do not understand every bit of this right now. This journal will help you practice gently, but effectively. Give yourself permission to not be perfect, so over time you can be your best in your sport, school, and whatever else you choose to take on.

WHAT'S IN YOUR A CIRCLE?

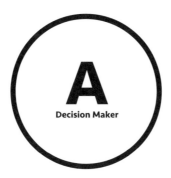

STEP 3 GOALS IN MOTION

Now that you have learned the strategies (ways you can manage your situations and your game) let's talk about goals. Goals are great! When you think of your goals do they get you excited? Do you feel pressure? Both? In this journal you will practice maximizing your ability to set and reach your goals.

GOAL BEYOND THE GOAL®

People can feel stuck, unmotivated, or be worried about a result. These are common issues when it comes to the mental side of the sport. A solution to these issues is having a goal beyond a goal.

Goal Beyond The Goal® is a strategy used to keep people mentally focused on what they want to do in the moment, to support their desired outcome. For example, I was working with a basketball player (I will call her Addison), who would always hesitate when she shot the basket, but she wanted to make more shots. She was worried about making a mistake, and did not want to be taken out of the game. When she would go up for a shot, she would tend to pass it off, or miss. She was mentally distracted or disconnected from her body because of those thoughts.

Addison had worry in her A Circle and it was controlling her. I asked her, "Addison, what do you want to have in your A Circle when you are shooting?" She said, "My form and how I shoot." Then I asked, "After you make the shot, then what do you want to be focusing on?" She said, "Defense and getting the ball back."

Acknowledging what was in her A Circle (worry and negative thoughts), replacing that with what she wanted in her A Circle (her form and technique), keeps her mind connected to her body. Giving her a new place to land (getting the ball back/defense), assures that she can stay connected through the process.

Without a new place to land (defense or getting the ball back), beyond the desired outcome (making the shot), people tend to mentally leave their body or bail out. It's important to have a Goal Beyond The Goal® mentality throughout your day to keep you moving forward toward your bigger goals. This will help you stay aligned with your behavior to achieve what you want daily.

Whenever you feel stagnant or unmotivated, use this strategy to support your process. If you're frustrated because you can't get a skill, focus on what you want to be doing after you learn the skill. It creates a window to move through, instead of a door that you're pounding your head against. Example: How do I want to hit the ball so that I can get to first base? Or what do I need to focus on while doing my giant to help me move into my flyaway?

Long-term Goal Beyond The Goal® mentality helps you understand how everything that you are going through now, easy or hard, is supporting what you want for yourself, in your future. For example, if I ask an athlete, "What is your goal in three years?" And they say, "To be in the Olympics." What we are doing is taking a snapshot of where they want to be three years down the road, throwing it into their time-line and dropping it down. **This aligns the athlete with what they want for themselves in the future, today.**

Moving forward, everything that they are doing today is helping them prepare to be successful for the Olympics tomorrow. Looking at it from this perspective gives them the ability to continue moving forward even on the rough days. It keeps their mentality **in the process** instead of worrying about every single daily result or outcome.

Think about where you want to be three years down the road. In this journal you will work toward all of your goals effectively, efficiently, and successfully.

STEP 4 STRATEGIES FOR SUCCESS

Do people ever tell you that you are "so talented"? Do you get frustrated and feel pressure when people talk about your talent or your potential? Would you like to be able to wrap your head around your own unconscious strategy for success?

This 4-question strategy gives you the ability to be aware of your own unconscious recipe for success — connect and practice this strategy in your behavior (in this case your sport) — connect it into your goals in the short-term and long-term.

Question 1: What is your goal beyond the goal?
We worked on this in Book 1. Think about your goal three years down the road. Where do you see yourself in three years? We are taking a snapshot of that, throwing it out into your timeline, and dropping it down. Practice acting, speaking, performing, and behaving from your goal's perspective. Your goal is seeking you as much as you are seeking it.

Question 2: What would be a good goal for you this season?
Set a goal six months out. Result goals are fine, as long as you are focusing on what you need to do to contribute to getting those results. For example: If I'm a volleyball player, I know that when I use the Learning Strategy®, I play my best. To achieve my six month goal I will focus on the Learning Strategy®. The result does not belong in your A Circle when you are practicing your sport or living your life. The result is ALWAYS a goal beyond the goal. FOCUS ON THE STRATEGY that works for YOU.

Question 3: What do you do well?
You can think about what you do well in your sport, or, what you do well in anything. What do people say that you do well? Are you good at mechanics or technique? Are you strong? Do you have good

timing? Think of situations where you were successful or confident — what were you doing well? Give yourself permission throughout this book to dig into what you do really well. Layer it, connect with it, and build on it!

Question 4: How are you doing it well?
Think of a situation where you were completely successful; it could have been yesterday or years ago. I want you to go back *into* that experience. Have that experience. Now, step out of that experience. How were you doing it well? Was it something that you said to yourself, something that you saw, something that you felt, something that you heard, or a combination? Did one come before the other or did they happen at the same time? Also, what was in your A Circle in that situation and what strategies were you using? *This is something I want you to practice.*

When you are doing this Strategy For Success, and in particular, answering question 4, how are you doing it well? Allow your mind to take you through the experience. There is no right or wrong in this process. The more you connect with what is happening unconsciously, the more you will be able to use it consciously.

I first experienced this process when I was 35. I was asked the question "Where in the past were you completely successful?" I went back to when I was eight years old. I was water skiing in a boat show. I was standing on the shoulders of two girls below me and three men below them. It was called the 3-2-1 pyramid. I remembered being completely successful. I could **feel** the people below me shaking because we were heavy, I could **see** the crowd cheering as I waved to them, I could **see** and **feel** and **hear** the water below us, and **I was saying to myself**..."This is so cool!" This was my recipe for success in that situation. *It was something I felt, saw, heard and said to myself, all at the same time.* I had myself in my A Circle and I was successful. It was amazing. Once you experience consciously what your success strategy was unconsciously and understand how to practice it moving forward, it becomes available to you. Similar to A-Circle®. You do not have to necessarily think about it for you to have the benefit of it. Make sense? Give yourself permission to not be perfect as you practice connecting these ideas, and your new awareness to your life. If you are having trouble wrapping your head around this completely right now, no worries! I am also available to support you with sessions one-on-one, or please ask me questions in the Facebook Group. The journal questions will be great practice as well!

POTENTIAL

What does is it mean to be able to tap into our potential?
We can practice living in our potential by understanding our own unconscious recipe for success. In Book 1, I mentioned that we all have strategies, and strategies are what we use to be successful or not successful. Typically, before Book 1, strategies were happening without conscious awareness. Book 1 taught us how to practice strategies with awareness. Now, in Book 2, we're adding more awareness to what was happening when we were successful. This awareness provides us the ability to connect our success to our goals.

The result is:
• Our mind and our body are on the same page.
• Our conscious mind and unconscious mind are congruent.
• Who we are (our being) and what we do (our behavior) are essentially connected.

This is when we are SO CONNECTED. When we live, perform, and behave from this perspective, we are performing in our full potential.

Now that you are aware of the strategy you used when you were successful, can you see how you can practice it more often? Can you see how you can use it to achieve your goals this season, and your goal beyond the goal? Can you see how you can use this strategy for success to support you in other areas of your life?

AWARENESS PROVIDES US THE ABILITY TO CONNECT OUR SUCCESS TO OUR GOALS.

© Stacey Herman Goodrich

STEP 5 PURGE IT. VENT. GET IT OUT!

Purge everything that you're thinking about, get it out. If you have an opportunity to vent do it, but make sure the person you're venting to understands that *you don't need to be fixed*. You're not broken and they don't need to interject themselves into your A Circle. You just want to talk and *get it out*!

Or —journal it. Acknowledging your feelings and writing them down is important. Once you move through the problem you will see more of the solution. Getting to the root of the problem is essential because that's where your solution lies.

After you get through the issues that you are feeling or experiencing —then what? Now what do you want to do? How do you want to use your situation to build on, to create more, and to be better because of it? For example, think about the one thing today that is completely bothering you. Now I want you to turn it around and be grateful for it. This is another opportunity to journal.

Experience the feelings that you are having; maybe you feel them in your body. If so, what part of your body? You can use color as well to express what's going on inside. Also, you may need to hear yourself process —just go on a walk and talk yourself through some things that you are experiencing or feeling. Practice taking your judgment of yourself out of your A Circle. The more accepting you can be of yourself, the more success you will have in becoming all that you want to be! Be gentle with yourself, but go after it!

YOU ARE READY TO DO THE WORK.
TRUST THE PROCESS.

WHAT DO YOU DO WELL? HOW ARE YOU DOING IT WELL?

PRACTICE THAT TO TAP INTO YOUR TALENT.

© Stacey Herman Goodrich

MONTH _____ 20 ____

MONDAY	TUESDAY	WEDNESDAY	THURSDAY

CONNECT who you are **TO** what you do.
Live in **YOUR POTENTIAL** one day at a time.

© Stacey Herman Goodrich

FRIDAY	SATURDAY	SUNDAY

week 1

MONDAY DAILY JOURNALING   DATE _____

MENTAL MINDSET FOR THE WEEK

Welcome to Book 2. The next three months will focus on you, your goals, and what you want. You create your reality.

JOURNALING PROMPTS

O Pick an intentional word or phrase of the day that is directly related to your goals. What do you want?

_____

O Think about moving forward. What do you want to have in your A Circle? How will that support you? Today, practice putting more of *you* into your A Circle to move toward your goals.

_____
_____
_____
_____
_____
_____

O Think about what went well and what did not go well in the past. What strategies were you using in those situations? What was in your A Circle?

_____
_____
_____
_____
_____
_____

MENTAL STRENGTH COACHING JOURNAL   33

○ How have your strategies evolved in the past three months? What are you more aware of? How have you been more accepting of yourself in your situation(s)?

_____

_____

_____

_____

_____

_____

○ What goals have you achieved in the last three months? What strategies did you use to support those goals?

_____

_____

_____

_____

_____

_____

○ What do you want to achieve in the next three months?

_____

_____

_____

_____

_____

_____

○ What has been in your way of achieving your goals in the past? What is something that you don't want people to know about you? What limiting beliefs do you have about yourself, or your life, or your situation(s)?

_____

_____

_____

_____

_____

_____

TUESDAY DAILY JOURNALING   DATE _____

JOURNALING PROMPTS

O Pick your intentional word or phrase of the day. Again, connect it directly to your goals.

_____

O How did yesterday's intentional word or phrase of the day support your goals? How can you support your goals more intentionally?

_____
_____
_____
_____

O What is your goal beyond the goal? Where do you want to be 3 years down the road?

_____
_____
_____
_____

O What is your goal for the next 3 months? What strategies do you use to support yourself in achieving your goals during these next 3 months?

_____
_____
_____
_____

MENTAL STRENGTH COACHING JOURNAL   35

O What do you do well? What do people say you do well? What are you good at in
   your sport and outside of your sport?

   _____

   _____

   _____

   _____

O Think of a situation where something went well. Go into that experience... and
   now step out of it. How were you doing that particular thing well? Was it something you saw? Something you felt? Something you said to yourself? Something
   you heard? Or a combination?

   _____

   _____

   _____

   _____

O This is your strategy for success. Can you use this more often? Where?

   _____

   _____

   _____

   _____

O Can you see how you can use this strategy to achieve your goals in the next 3
   months? In the next 3 years? How could you have used it this past week?

   _____

   _____

   _____

   _____

O What inspired you today?

   _____

   _____

   _____

   _____

WEDNESDAY DAILY JOURNALING   DATE _____

JOURNALING PROMPTS

O Pick your intentional word or phrase of the day.

_____

O How has the intentional word of the day changed how you live your life?

_____

_____

O Do you like to see your way through your skills/plays/sport? Or feel your way
through, think your way through, talk your way through, or a combination?

_____

_____

_____

O Think of a time when you were successful. What strategy were you using? What
was in your A Circle?

_____

_____

_____

O Can you practice using this strategy moving forward? In what past situations could
you have used this strategy? With coaches? Teammates?

_____

_____

_____

O Really dig down deep to think about what you do well. What gifts do you have that
you can become more aware of? I want you to think about where things went really
well in the past. How did you contribute to that?

_____

_____

_____

O I am so proud of you. Get comfortable in your success. Know that you always have more to grow and do. BUT, get comfortable in it! We do not have to struggle to be more successful. Where in the past did you sabotage your success or yourself?

_____

_____

_____

_____

O Now, think about how you could have taken care of yourself better in those situations. Could you have gotten stronger without the injury? Could you have been better without struggling for the entire season?

_____

_____

_____

O Do you seek support from outside of yourself or inside of yourself? What works best for you? Do THAT more often. What ever works for you is great. Understanding what you need is what you can practice more.

_____

_____

_____

O Think about your situation. What are some great things about your situation (coaches...team...parents...club...school) that can support you to achieve your goals?

_____

_____

_____

O Outside of your sport —what do you love?

_____

_____

_____

_____

THURSDAY DAILY JOURNALING   DATE _____

JOURNALING PROMPTS

O What is your intentional word of the day? Pick one that directly connects you to your gift!

_____

O Remember that you have a "present self "and a "goal self." Practice stepping out of your "present self" and stepping into your "goal self " more often. Add your ability to share your gift with the world more often. What do you do well and how do you do it well? How can you explore ways to do and be more of that??

_____
_____
_____
_____

O Do you have situations where your A Circle gets crowded with negative thoughts, or negative energy, or negative people? Are you having trouble kicking them out? If you are struggling with negative things in your A Circle, how can you replace them? Do you want to?

_____
_____
_____
_____

O For example, if you have fear/anxiety/worry in your A Circle, it is only there to help you pay attention, to think about what you want to be doing, or to remind yourself to focus on what you are doing physically. Practice thanking — yes thanking — that energy so you can use it to your advantage. Practice thanking _old_ situations as well. What could you have done to support yourself better in the past?

_____
_____
_____

MENTAL STRENGTH COACHING JOURNAL   39

O Think of some goals outside of your sport that you want to achieve. List them.

O Can you see how adding more of yourself to your goals outside of your sport adds
   more to your goals? How?

O We can only give away what we have inside ourselves. The great thing is that it will
   never take from us to support others when we have it for ourselves first. What do
   you see in others? If it is ugliness then love yourself more :)

I AM SO PROUD OF YOU!

FRIDAY DAILY JOURNALING   DATE _____

JOURNALING PROMPTS

O Pick your intentional word or phrase of the day. Think about your week. What can you focus on today that will support your entire week?

_____

O Can you think of situations this week where you were more in your own A Circle?

_____
_____
_____
_____

O How was that helpful for you?

_____
_____
_____
_____

O When you think about your A Circle, can you see how your ability to manage it can be helpful for your goals? What did you learn this week about how you are able to manage your A Circle?

_____
_____
_____
_____

O Think of situations in the past that did not go well. An injury? Maybe you broke down under pressure, or you were worried about what people were thinking of you. Write them down.

_____
_____
_____
_____

MENTAL STRENGTH COACHING JOURNAL   41

O Looking back, do you see that if you would have known these tools and strategies, they would have been helpful? Remember, you did the best you could with what you knew at the time. What strategies could you have used? What could you have had in your A Circle?

O This week, when you look back, name 3 reasons for your success.

O What do you do well? How do you do it well? Remember: nobody does your skills/ sport/game better than you —be confident in that.

O Step back and practice joy. Where do you have the most joy in your life? Do more of that.

SATURDAY DAILY JOURNALING   DATE _____

CELEBRATION DAY!

O Think of 5 situations where you were successful. Write them down.

_____

_____

_____

_____

_____

_____

O Think of 5 things that you accomplished this week. Write them down.

_____

_____

_____

_____

_____

_____

O Where did you build strength this week mentally? Physically?

_____

_____

_____

_____

_____

_____

O What did you learn from this week that can support you to achieve your goals?

_____

_____

_____

_____

_____

_____

O What went well? What didn't go well? And what can you learn from both?

O Remember that you are not equal to the result. When you accomplish a goal, it is fantastic —*but you are not equal to it.* Learn from it so you can use that experience and same strategy to build success. Where this week can you use this?

O Also, you are not equal to the mistake, or what did not go well. Separate yourself from those situations so that you can also learn from them. Can you think of any situation this week where you can practice this? Are you hard on yourself? Do you have high expectations of yourself? That's okay, but neither of those things belong in your A Circle when you are doing your sport. Did you have situations this week where this got in your way?

SUNDAY! DAILY JOURNALING   DATE _____

DREAM DAY!

○ Give yourself permission to dream. We need to practice dreaming. It's not a bad thing to desire, or to want things in your life! Putting your best self into your life, sharing your gift to the world, being more of you, is your responsibility and your job. Dreaming only inspires more of you in that way. As you practice putting more of you into your life, you can share that with others; that is inspiring. Where this week were you more of you?

_____

_____

_____

_____

_____

○ Regarding your answer above, were people receptive to it or a little bit threatened?

_____

_____

Remember this: I can only see in you what I have in myself. So, if I don't see you in all your brightness, it's not because something is wrong with *you*. It is *my* lack that is the issue. Do not let someone else's inability to see your light dim it. Practice being your light. Practice seeing other's light as well.

_____

_____

_____

_____

_____

_____

PRACTICE THESE 10 MINDSET RULES:

1 Set big, bold, tremendous goals.

2 Be grateful for everything you have today, and everything you don't have yet.

3 Be 100% accountable for your life. It doesn't mean that everything is your fault, but taking 100% responsibility for it moves you forward with strength.

4 Be thankful – for everything that went well and for everything that didn't go well.

5 Act, speak, think, and perform from the perspective of your Goal Beyond The Goal®.

6 Replace every negative thought with positive thought.

7 Add enthusiasm, energy and certainty to everything in your life!

8 Disregard disempowering actions and language.

9 There are no problems, only opportunities.

10 Bring the data, not the drama!

week 2

MONDAY DAILY JOURNALING   DATE _____

MENTAL MINDSET FOR THE WEEK

Isn't it great to go from a lack mentality to performing your best? Congratulations on shifting your mindset.

JOURNALING PROMPTS

○ Pick an intentional word or phrase of the day that is directly related to your goals. What do you want?

_____

○ Think about moving forward. What do you want to have in your A Circle? How will that support you? Today, practice putting more of *you* into your A Circle to move toward your goals.

_____
_____
_____
_____
_____
_____

○ Think about what went well and what did not go well in the past. What strategies were you using in those situations? What was in your A Circle?

_____
_____
_____
_____
_____
_____

MENTAL STRENGTH COACHING JOURNAL   47

O How have your strategies evolved in the past three months? What are you more aware of? How have you been more accepting of yourself in your situation(s)?

O What goals have you achieved in the last three months? What strategies did you use to support those goals?

O What do you want to achieve in the next three months?

O What has been in your way of achieving your goals in the past? What is something that you don't want people to know about you? What limiting beliefs do you have about yourself, or your life, or your situation(s)?

TUESDAY DAILY JOURNALING   DATE _____

JOURNALING PROMPTS

O Pick your intentional word or phrase of the day. Again, connect it directly to
your goals.

_____

O How did yesterday's intentional word or phrase of the day support your goals?
How can you support your goals more intentionally?

_____
_____
_____
_____
_____

O What is your goal beyond the goal? Where do you want to be 3 years down
the road?

_____
_____
_____
_____
_____

O What is your goal for the next 3 months? What strategies do you use to support
yourself in achieving your goals during these next 3 months?

_____
_____
_____
_____

O What do you do well? What do people say you do well? What are you good at in your sport and outside of your sport?

_____

_____

_____

_____

O Think of a situation where something went well. Go into that experience... and now step out of it. How were you doing that particular thing well? Was it something you saw? Something you felt? Something you said to yourself? Something you heard? Or a combination?

_____

_____

_____

_____

O This is your strategy for success. Can you use this more often? Where?

_____

_____

_____

_____

O Can you see how you can use this strategy to achieve your goals in the next 3 months? In the next 3 years? How could you have used it this past week?

_____

_____

_____

_____

O What inspired you today?

_____

_____

_____

_____

WEDNESDAY DAILY JOURNALING   DATE _____

JOURNALING PROMPTS

○ Pick your intentional word or phrase of the day.

_____

○ How has the intentional word of the day changed how you live your life?

_____

_____

○ Do you like to see your way through your skills/plays/sport? Or feel your way
   through, think your way through, talk your way through, or a combination?

_____

_____

_____

○ Think of a time when you were successful. What strategy were you using? What
   was in your A Circle?

_____

_____

_____

○ Can you practice using this strategy moving forward? In what past situations could
   you have used this strategy? With coaches? Teammates?

_____

_____

_____

○ Really dig down deep to think about what you do well. What gifts do you have that
   you can become more aware of? I want you to think about where things went really
   well in the past. How did you contribute to that?

_____

_____

_____

○ I am so proud of you. Get comfortable in your success. Know that you always have more to grow and do. BUT, get comfortable in it! We do not have to struggle to be more successful. Where in the past did you sabotage your success or yourself?

○ Now, think about how you could have taken care of yourself better in those situations. Could you have gotten stronger without the injury? Could you have been better without struggling for the entire season?

○ Do you seek support from outside of yourself or inside of yourself? What works best for you? Do THAT more often. What ever works for you is great. Understanding what you need is what you can practice more.

○ Think about your situation. What are some great things about your situation (coaches...team...parents...club...school) that can support you to achieve your goals?

○ Outside of your sport —what do you love?

THURSDAY DAILY JOURNALING   DATE _____

JOURNALING PROMPTS

O What is your intentional word of the day? Pick one that directly connects you to
your gift!

_____

O Remember that you have a "present self "and a "goal self." Practice stepping out of
your "present self" and stepping into your "goal self " more often. Add your ability
to share your gift with the world more often. What do you do well and how do you
do it well? How can you explore ways to do and be more of that??

_____

_____

_____

_____

O Do you have situations where your A Circle gets crowded with negative thoughts,
or negative energy, or negative people? Are you having trouble kicking them out?
If you are struggling with negative things in your A Circle, how can you replace
them? Do you want to?

_____

_____

_____

_____

O For example, if you have fear/anxiety/worry in your A Circle, it is only there to help
you pay attention, to think about what you want to be doing, or to remind yourself
to focus on what you are doing physically. Practice thanking — yes thanking — that
energy so you can use it to your advantage. Practice thanking *old* situations as
well. What could you have done to support yourself better in the past?

_____

_____

_____

_____

MENTAL STRENGTH COACHING JOURNAL   53

O Think of some goals outside of your sport that you want to achieve. List them.

O Can you see how adding more of yourself to your goals outside of your sport adds more to your goals? How?

O We can only give away what we have inside ourselves. The great thing is that it will never take from us to support others when we have it for ourselves first. What do you see in others? If it is ugliness then love yourself more :)

I AM SO PROUD OF YOU!

FRIDAY DAILY JOURNALING   DATE _____

JOURNALING PROMPTS

O Pick your intentional word or phrase of the day. Think about your week. What can
   you focus on today that will support your entire week?

   _____

O Can you think of situations this week where you were more in your own A Circle?

   _____
   _____
   _____
   _____

O How was that helpful for you?

   _____
   _____
   _____
   _____

O When you think about your A Circle, can you see how your ability to manage it can
   be helpful for your goals? What did you learn this week about how you are able to
   manage your A Circle?

   _____
   _____
   _____
   _____

O Think of situations in the past that did not go well. An injury? Maybe you broke
   down under pressure, or you were worried about what people were thinking of
   you. Write them down.

   _____
   _____
   _____
   _____

O Looking back, do you see that if you would have known these tools and strategies, they would have been helpful? Remember, you did the best you could with what you knew at the time. What strategies could you have used? What could you have had in your A Circle?

_____
_____
_____
_____
_____

O This week, when you look back, name 3 reasons for your success.

_____
_____
_____
_____
_____
_____

O What do you do well? How do you do it well? Remember: nobody does your skills/ sport/game better than you —be confident in that.

_____
_____
_____
_____
_____
_____

O Step back and practice joy. Where do you have the most joy in your life? Do more of that.

_____
_____
_____
_____
_____

SATURDAY DAILY JOURNALING   DATE _____

CELEBRATION DAY!

O Think of 5 situations where you were successful. Write them down.

_____
_____
_____
_____
_____
_____

O Think of 5 things that you accomplished this week. Write them down.

_____
_____
_____
_____
_____
_____

O Where did you build strength this week mentally? Physically?

_____
_____
_____
_____
_____
_____

O What did you learn from this week that can support you to achieve your goals?

_____
_____
_____
_____
_____

O What went well? What didn't go well? And what can you learn from both?

O Remember that you are not equal to the result. When you accomplish a goal, it is fantastic —*but you are not equal to it.* Learn from it so you can use that experience and same strategy to build success. Where this week can you use this?

O Also, you are not equal to the mistake, or what did not go well. Separate yourself from those situations so that you can also learn from them. Can you think of any situation this week where you can practice this? Are you hard on yourself? Do you have high expectations of yourself? That's okay, but neither of those things belong in your A Circle when you are doing your sport. Did you have situations this week where this got in your way?

SUNDAY! DAILY JOURNALING   DATE _____

DREAM DAY!

O Give yourself permission to dream. We need to practice dreaming. It's not a bad thing to desire, or to want things in your life! Putting your best self into your life, sharing your gift to the world, being more of you, is your responsibility and your job. Dreaming only inspires more of you in that way. As you practice putting more of you into your life, you can share that with others; that is inspiring. Where this week were you more of you?

_____

_____

_____

_____

_____

O Regarding your answer above, were people receptive to it or a little bit threatened?

_____

_____

_____

Remember this: I can only see in you what I have in myself. So, if I don't see you in all your brightness, it's not because something is wrong with *you*. It is *my* lack that is the issue. Do not let someone else's inability to see your light dim it. Practice being your light. Practice seeing other's light as well.

_____

_____

_____

_____

_____

_____

PRACTICE THESE 10 MINDSET RULES:

1 Set big, bold, tremendous goals.

2 Be grateful for everything you have today, and everything you don't have yet.

3 Be 100% accountable for your life. It doesn't mean that everything is your fault, but taking 100% responsibility for it moves you forward with strength.

4 Be thankful – for everything that went well and for everything that didn't go well.

5 Act, speak, think, and perform from the perspective of your Goal Beyond The Goal®.

6 Replace every negative thought with positive thought.

7 Add enthusiasm, energy and certainty to everything in your life!

8 Disregard disempowering actions and language.

9 There are no problems, only opportunities.

10 Bring the data, not the drama!

week 3

MONDAY DAILY JOURNALING   DATE _____

MENTAL MINDSET FOR THE WEEK

As you are more accepting of yourself in your own A Circle, how does this acceptance reward you?

JOURNALING PROMPTS

O Pick an intentional word or phrase of the day that is directly related to your goals. What do you want?

_____

O Think about moving forward. What do you want to have in your A Circle? How will that support you? Today, practice putting more of *you* into your A Circle to move toward your goals.

_____
_____
_____
_____
_____
_____

O Think about what went well and what did not go well in the past. What strategies were you using in those situations? What was in your A Circle?

_____
_____
_____
_____
_____
_____

O How have your strategies evolved in the past three months? What are you more aware of? How have you been more accepting of yourself in your situation(s)?

O What goals have you achieved in the last three months? What strategies did you use to support those goals?

O What do you want to achieve in the next three months?

O What has been in your way of achieving your goals in the past? What is something that you don't want people to know about you? What limiting beliefs do you have about yourself, or your life, or your situation(s)?

TUESDAY DAILY JOURNALING   DATE _____

JOURNALING PROMPTS

○ Pick your intentional word or phrase of the day. Again, connect it directly to your goals.

_____

○ How did yesterday's intentional word or phrase of the day support your goals? How can you support your goals more intentionally?

_____
_____
_____
_____

○ What is your goal beyond the goal? Where do you want to be 3 years down the road?

_____
_____
_____
_____

○ What is your goal for the next 3 months? What strategies do you use to support yourself in achieving your goals during these next 3 months?

_____
_____
_____
_____

MENTAL STRENGTH COACHING JOURNAL 63

O What do you do well? What do people say you do well? What are you good at in your sport and outside of your sport?

O Think of a situation where something went well. Go into that experience... and now step out of it. How were you doing that particular thing well? Was it something you saw? Something you felt? Something you said to yourself? Something you heard? Or a combination?

O This is your strategy for success. Can you use this more often? Where?

O Can you see how you can use this strategy to achieve your goals in the next 3 months? In the next 3 years? How could you have used it this past week?

O What inspired you today?

WEDNESDAY DAILY JOURNALING   DATE _____

JOURNALING PROMPTS

O Pick your intentional word or phrase of the day.

_____

O How has the intentional word of the day changed how you live your life?

_____

_____

O Do you like to see your way through your skills/plays/sport? Or feel your way
through, think your way through, talk your way through, or a combination?

_____

_____

_____

O Think of a time when you were successful. What strategy were you using? What
was in your A Circle?

_____

_____

_____

O Can you practice using this strategy moving forward? In what past situations could
you have used this strategy? With coaches? Teammates?

_____

_____

_____

O Really dig down deep to think about what you do well. What gifts do you have that
you can become more aware of? I want you to think about where things went really
well in the past. How did you contribute to that?

_____

_____

_____

MENTAL STRENGTH COACHING JOURNAL   65

O I am so proud of you. Get comfortable in your success. Know that you always have
   more to grow and do. BUT, get comfortable in it! We do not have to struggle to be
   more successful. Where in the past did you sabotage your success or yourself?

_____

_____

_____

_____

O Now, think about how you could have taken care of yourself better in those situations. Could you have gotten stronger without the injury? Could you have been
   better without struggling for the entire season?

_____

_____

_____

O Do you seek support from outside of yourself or inside of yourself? What works
   best for you? Do THAT more often. What ever works for you is great. Understanding what you need is what you can practice more.

_____

_____

_____

O Think about your situation. What are some great things about your situation
   (coaches...team...parents...club...school) that can support you to achieve
   your goals?

_____

_____

_____

O Outside of your sport —what do you love?

_____

_____

_____

_____

_____

THURSDAY DAILY JOURNALING   DATE _____

JOURNALING PROMPTS

O What is your intentional word of the day? Pick one that directly connects you to your gift!

_____

O Remember that you have a "present self "and a "goal self." Practice stepping out of your "present self" and stepping into your "goal self " more often. Add your ability to share your gift with the world more often. What do you do well and how do you do it well? How can you explore ways to do and be more of that??

_____
_____
_____
_____

O Do you have situations where your A Circle gets crowded with negative thoughts, or negative energy, or negative people? Are you having trouble kicking them out? If you are struggling with negative things in your A Circle, how can you replace them? Do you want to?

_____
_____
_____
_____

O For example, if you have fear/anxiety/worry in your A Circle, it is only there to help you pay attention, to think about what you want to be doing, or to remind yourself to focus on what you are doing physically. Practice thanking — yes thanking — that energy so you can use it to your advantage. Practice thanking *old* situations as well. What could you have done to support yourself better in the past?

_____
_____
_____
_____

O Think of some goals outside of your sport that you want to achieve. List them.

O Can you see how adding more of yourself to your goals outside of your sport adds more to your goals? How?

O We can only give away what we have inside ourselves. The great thing is that it will never take from us to support others when we have it for ourselves first. What do you see in others? If it is ugliness then love yourself more :)

I AM SO PROUD OF YOU!

FRIDAY DAILY JOURNALING   DATE _____

JOURNALING PROMPTS

O Pick your intentional word or phrase of the day. Think about your week. What can you focus on today that will support your entire week?

_____

O Can you think of situations this week where you were more in your own A Circle?

_____
_____
_____
_____

O How was that helpful for you?

_____
_____
_____
_____

O When you think about your A Circle, can you see how your ability to manage it can be helpful for your goals? What did you learn this week about how you are able to manage your A Circle?

_____
_____
_____
_____

O Think of situations in the past that did not go well. An injury? Maybe you broke down under pressure, or you were worried about what people were thinking of you. Write them down.

_____
_____
_____
_____

O Looking back, do you see that if you would have known these tools and strategies, they would have been helpful? Remember, you did the best you could with what you knew at the time. What strategies could you have used? What could you have had in your A Circle?

O This week, when you look back, name 3 reasons for your success.

O What do you do well? How do you do it well? Remember: nobody does your skills/sport/game better than you —be confident in that.

O Step back and practice joy. Where do you have the most joy in your life? Do more of that.

SATURDAY DAILY JOURNALING   DATE _____

CELEBRATION DAY!

O Think of 5 situations where you were successful. Write them down.

_____

_____

_____

_____

_____

_____

O Think of 5 things that you accomplished this week. Write them down.

_____

_____

_____

_____

_____

_____

O Where did you build strength this week mentally? Physically?

_____

_____

_____

_____

_____

_____

O What did you learn from this week that can support you to achieve your goals?

_____

_____

_____

_____

_____

_____

O What went well? What didn't go well? And what can you learn from both?

O Remember that you are not equal to the result. When you accomplish a goal, it is fantastic —*but you are not equal to it.* Learn from it so you can use that experience and same strategy to build success. Where this week can you use this?

O Also, you are not equal to the mistake, or what did not go well. Separate yourself from those situations so that you can also learn from them. Can you think of any situation this week where you can practice this? Are you hard on yourself? Do you have high expectations of yourself? That's okay, but neither of those things belong in your A Circle when you are doing your sport. Did you have situations this week where this got in your way?

SUNDAY! DAILY JOURNALING   DATE _____

DREAM DAY!

O Give yourself permission to dream. We need to practice dreaming. It's not a bad
thing to desire, or to want things in your life! Putting your best self into your life,
sharing your gift to the world, being more of you, is your responsibility and your
job. Dreaming only inspires more of you in that way. As you practice putting more
of you into your life, you can share that with others; that is inspiring. Where this
week were you more of you?

_____

_____

_____

_____

_____

O Regarding your answer above, were people receptive to it or a little bit threatened?

_____

_____

_____

Remember this: I can only see in you what I have in myself. So, if I
don't see you in all your brightness, it's not because something is
wrong with *you*. It is *my* lack that is the issue. Do not let someone
else's inability to see your light dim it. Practice being your light.
Practice seeing other's light as well.

_____

_____

_____

_____

_____

_____

PRACTICE THESE 10 MINDSET RULES:

1 Set big, bold, tremendous goals.

2 Be grateful for everything you have today, and everything you don't have yet.

3 Be 100% accountable for your life. It doesn't mean that everything is your fault, but taking 100% responsibility for it moves you forward with strength.

4 Be thankful – for everything that went well and for everything that didn't go well.

5 Act, speak, think, and perform from the perspective of your Goal Beyond The Goal®.

6 Replace every negative thought with positive thought.

7 Add enthusiasm, energy and certainty to everything in your life!

8 Disregard disempowering actions and language.

9 There are no problems, only opportunities.

10 Bring the data, not the drama!

week 4

MONDAY DAILY JOURNALING   DATE _____

MENTAL MINDSET FOR THE WEEK

I like it that you are hard on yourself, or stubborn, or want to be better. However, make sure you are in control of these ideas, instead of your ideas controlling you.

JOURNALING PROMPTS

O Pick an intentional word or phrase of the day that is directly related to your goals. What do you want?

_____

O Think about moving forward. What do you want to have in your A Circle? How will that support you? Today, practice putting more of *you* into your A Circle to move toward your goals.

_____
_____
_____
_____
_____
_____

O Think about what went well and what did not go well in the past. What strategies were you using in those situations? What was in your A Circle?

_____
_____
_____
_____
_____
_____

MENTAL STRENGTH COACHING JOURNAL   75

O How have your strategies evolved in the past three months? What are you more aware of? How have you been more accepting of yourself in your situation(s)?

O What goals have you achieved in the last three months? What strategies did you use to support those goals?

O What do you want to achieve in the next three months?

O What has been in your way of achieving your goals in the past? What is something that you don't want people to know about you? What limiting beliefs do you have about yourself, or your life, or your situation(s)?

TUESDAY DAILY JOURNALING   DATE _____

JOURNALING PROMPTS

O Pick your intentional word or phrase of the day. Again, connect it directly to your goals.

_____

O How did yesterday's intentional word or phrase of the day support your goals? How can you support your goals more intentionally?

_____
_____
_____
_____
_____

O What is your goal beyond the goal? Where do you want to be 3 years down the road?

_____
_____
_____
_____
_____

O What is your goal for the next 3 months? What strategies do you use to support yourself in achieving your goals during these next 3 months?

_____
_____
_____
_____

MENTAL STRENGTH COACHING JOURNAL   77

O What do you do well? What do people say you do well? What are you good at in
   your sport and outside of your sport?

O Think of a situation where something went well. Go into that experience... and
   now step out of it. How were you doing that particular thing well? Was it something you saw? Something you felt? Something you said to yourself? Something
   you heard? Or a combination?

O This is your strategy for success. Can you use this more often? Where?

O Can you see how you can use this strategy to achieve your goals in the next 3
   months? In the next 3 years? How could you have used it this past week?

O What inspired you today?

WEDNESDAY DAILY JOURNALING   DATE _____

JOURNALING PROMPTS

O Pick your intentional word or phrase of the day.

_____

O How has the intentional word of the day changed how you live your life?

_____

_____

O Do you like to see your way through your skills/plays/sport? Or feel your way through, think your way through, talk your way through, or a combination?

_____

_____

_____

O Think of a time when you were successful. What strategy were you using? What was in your A Circle?

_____

_____

_____

O Can you practice using this strategy moving forward? In what past situations could you have used this strategy? With coaches? Teammates?

_____

_____

_____

O Really dig down deep to think about what you do well. What gifts do you have that you can become more aware of? I want you to think about where things went really well in the past. How did you contribute to that?

_____

_____

_____

O I am so proud of you. Get comfortable in your success. Know that you always have more to grow and do. BUT, get comfortable in it! We do not have to struggle to be more successful. Where in the past did you sabotage your success or yourself?

O Now, think about how you could have taken care of yourself better in those situations. Could you have gotten stronger without the injury? Could you have been better without struggling for the entire season?

O Do you seek support from outside of yourself or inside of yourself? What works best for you? Do THAT more often. What ever works for you is great. Understanding what you need is what you can practice more.

O Think about your situation. What are some great things about your situation (coaches...team...parents...club...school) that can support you to achieve your goals?

O Outside of your sport —what do you love?

THURSDAY DAILY JOURNALING   DATE _____

JOURNALING PROMPTS

O What is your intentional word of the day? Pick one that directly connects you to your gift!

_____

O Remember that you have a "present self "and a "goal self." Practice stepping out of your "present self" and stepping into your "goal self " more often. Add your ability to share your gift with the world more often. What do you do well and how do you do it well? How can you explore ways to do and be more of that??

_____

_____

_____

_____

O Do you have situations where your A Circle gets crowded with negative thoughts, or negative energy, or negative people? Are you having trouble kicking them out? If you are struggling with negative things in your A Circle, how can you replace them? Do you want to?

_____

_____

_____

_____

O For example, if you have fear/anxiety/worry in your A Circle, it is only there to help you pay attention, to think about what you want to be doing, or to remind yourself to focus on what you are doing physically. Practice thanking — yes thanking — that energy so you can use it to your advantage. Practice thanking *old* situations as well. What could you have done to support yourself better in the past?

_____

_____

_____

_____

O Think of some goals outside of your sport that you want to achieve. List them.

O Can you see how adding more of yourself to your goals outside of your sport adds more to your goals? How?

O We can only give away what we have inside ourselves. The great thing is that it will never take from us to support others when we have it for ourselves first. What do you see in others? If it is ugliness then love yourself more :)

I AM SO PROUD OF YOU!

FRIDAY DAILY JOURNALING   DATE _____

JOURNALING PROMPTS

O Pick your intentional word or phrase of the day. Think about your week. What can you focus on today that will support your entire week?

_____

O Can you think of situations this week where you were more in your own A Circle?

_____
_____
_____
_____

O How was that helpful for you?

_____
_____
_____
_____

O When you think about your A Circle, can you see how your ability to manage it can be helpful for your goals? What did you learn this week about how you are able to manage your A Circle?

_____
_____
_____
_____

O Think of situations in the past that did not go well. An injury? Maybe you broke down under pressure, or you were worried about what people were thinking of you. Write them down.

_____
_____
_____
_____

○ Looking back, do you see that if you would have known these tools and strategies, they would have been helpful? Remember, you did the best you could with what you knew at the time. What strategies could you have used? What could you have had in your A Circle?

○ This week, when you look back, name 3 reasons for your success.

○ What do you do well? How do you do it well? Remember: nobody does your skills/sport/game better than you —be confident in that.

○ Step back and practice joy. Where do you have the most joy in your life? Do more of that.

SATURDAY DAILY JOURNALING   DATE _____

CELEBRATION DAY!

O Think of 5 situations where you were successful. Write them down.

_____
_____
_____
_____
_____
_____

O Think of 5 things that you accomplished this week. Write them down.

_____
_____
_____
_____
_____
_____

O Where did you build strength this week mentally? Physically?

_____
_____
_____
_____
_____
_____

O What did you learn from this week that can support you to achieve your goals?

_____
_____
_____
_____
_____
_____

O What went well? What didn't go well? And what can you learn from both?

O Remember that you are not equal to the result. When you accomplish a goal, it is fantastic —*but you are not equal to it.* Learn from it so you can use that experience and same strategy to build success. Where this week can you use this?

O Also, you are not equal to the mistake, or what did not go well. Separate yourself from those situations so that you can also learn from them. Can you think of any situation this week where you can practice this? Are you hard on yourself? Do you have high expectations of yourself? That's okay, but neither of those things belong in your A Circle when you are doing your sport. Did you have situations this week where this got in your way?

SUNDAY! DAILY JOURNALING   DATE _____

DREAM DAY!

O Give yourself permission to dream. We need to practice dreaming. It's not a bad thing to desire, or to want things in your life! Putting your best self into your life, sharing your gift to the world, being more of you, is your responsibility and your job. Dreaming only inspires more of you in that way. As you practice putting more of you into your life, you can share that with others; that is inspiring. Where this week were you more of you?

_____

_____

_____

_____

_____

O Regarding your answer above, were people receptive to it or a little bit threatened?

_____

_____

_____

Remember this: I can only see in you what I have in myself. So, if I don't see you in all your brightness, it's not because something is wrong with *you*. It is *my* lack that is the issue. Do not let someone else's inability to see your light dim it. Practice being your light. Practice seeing other's light as well.

_____

_____

_____

_____

_____

_____

_____

PRACTICE THESE 10 MINDSET RULES:

1 Set big, bold, tremendous goals.

2 Be grateful for everything you have today, and everything you don't have yet.

3 Be 100% accountable for your life. It doesn't mean that everything is your fault, but taking 100% responsibility for it moves you forward with strength.

4 Be thankful – for everything that went well and for everything that didn't go well.

5 Act, speak, think, and perform from the perspective of your Goal Beyond The Goal®.

6 Replace every negative thought with positive thought.

7 Add enthusiasm, energy and certainty to everything in your life!

8 Disregard disempowering actions and language.

9 There are no problems, only opportunities.

10 Bring the data, not the drama!

week 5

MONDAY DAILY JOURNALING   DATE _____

MENTAL MINDSET FOR THE WEEK

Practice stretching yourself through the ideas presented in this book. This is not about being perfect today; it's about using these strategies to be your best tomorrow.

JOURNALING PROMPTS

O Pick an intentional word or phrase of the day that is directly related to your goals. What do you want?

_____

O Think about moving forward. What do you want to have in your A Circle? How will that support you? Today, practice putting more of *you* into your A Circle to move toward your goals.

_____
_____
_____
_____
_____
_____

O Think about what went well and what did not go well in the past. What strategies were you using in those situations? What was in your A Circle?

_____
_____
_____
_____
_____
_____

MENTAL STRENGTH COACHING JOURNAL   89

O How have your strategies evolved in the past three months? What are you more
   aware of? How have you been more accepting of yourself in your situation(s)?

_____

_____

_____

_____

_____

_____

O What goals have you achieved in the last three months? What strategies did you
   use to support those goals?

_____

_____

_____

_____

_____

O What do you want to achieve in the next three months?

_____

_____

_____

_____

_____

O What has been in your way of achieving your goals in the past? What is something
   that you don't want people to know about you? What limiting beliefs do you have
   about yourself, or your life, or your situation(s)?

_____

_____

_____

_____

_____

TUESDAY DAILY JOURNALING   DATE _____

JOURNALING PROMPTS

O Pick your intentional word or phrase of the day. Again, connect it directly to your goals.

_____

O How did yesterday's intentional word or phrase of the day support your goals? How can you support your goals more intentionally?

_____
_____
_____
_____
_____

O What is your goal beyond the goal? Where do you want to be 3 years down the road?

_____
_____
_____
_____
_____

O What is your goal for the next 3 months? What strategies do you use to support yourself in achieving your goals during these next 3 months?

_____
_____
_____
_____

MENTAL STRENGTH COACHING JOURNAL   91

O What do you do well? What do people say you do well? What are you good at in
   your sport and outside of your sport?

   _____

   _____

   _____

   _____

O Think of a situation where something went well. Go into that experience... and
   now step out of it. How were you doing that particular thing well? Was it something you saw? Something you felt? Something you said to yourself? Something
   you heard? Or a combination?

   _____

   _____

   _____

   _____

O This is your strategy for success. Can you use this more often? Where?

   _____

   _____

   _____

   _____

O Can you see how you can use this strategy to achieve your goals in the next 3
   months? In the next 3 years? How could you have used it this past week?

   _____

   _____

   _____

   _____

O What inspired you today?

   _____

   _____

   _____

   _____

WEDNESDAY DAILY JOURNALING   DATE _____

JOURNALING PROMPTS

O Pick your intentional word or phrase of the day.

_____

O How has the intentional word of the day changed how you live your life?

_____

_____

O Do you like to see your way through your skills/plays/sport? Or feel your way through, think your way through, talk your way through, or a combination?

_____

_____

_____

O Think of a time when you were successful. What strategy were you using? What was in your A Circle?

_____

_____

_____

O Can you practice using this strategy moving forward? In what past situations could you have used this strategy? With coaches? Teammates?

_____

_____

_____

O Really dig down deep to think about what you do well. What gifts do you have that you can become more aware of? I want you to think about where things went really well in the past. How did you contribute to that?

_____

_____

_____

○ I am so proud of you. Get comfortable in your success. Know that you always have more to grow and do. BUT, get comfortable in it! We do not have to struggle to be more successful. Where in the past did you sabotage your success or yourself?

_____

_____

_____

_____

○ Now, think about how you could have taken care of yourself better in those situations. Could you have gotten stronger without the injury? Could you have been better without struggling for the entire season?

_____

_____

_____

○ Do you seek support from outside of yourself or inside of yourself? What works best for you? Do THAT more often. What ever works for you is great. Understanding what you need is what you can practice more.

_____

_____

_____

○ Think about your situation. What are some great things about your situation (coaches...team...parents...club...school) that can support you to achieve your goals?

_____

_____

_____

○ Outside of your sport —what do you love?

_____

_____

_____

_____

THURSDAY DAILY JOURNALING   DATE _____

JOURNALING PROMPTS

O What is your intentional word of the day? Pick one that directly connects you to your gift!

_____

O Remember that you have a "present self "and a "goal self." Practice stepping out of your "present self" and stepping into your "goal self " more often. Add your ability to share your gift with the world more often. What do you do well and how do you do it well? How can you explore ways to do and be more of that??

_____

_____

_____

_____

O Do you have situations where your A Circle gets crowded with negative thoughts, or negative energy, or negative people? Are you having trouble kicking them out? If you are struggling with negative things in your A Circle, how can you replace them? Do you want to?

_____

_____

_____

_____

O For example, if you have fear/anxiety/worry in your A Circle, it is only there to help you pay attention, to think about what you want to be doing, or to remind yourself to focus on what you are doing physically. Practice thanking — yes thanking — that energy so you can use it to your advantage. Practice thanking *old* situations as well. What could you have done to support yourself better in the past?

_____

_____

_____

O Think of some goals outside of your sport that you want to achieve. List them.

O Can you see how adding more of yourself to your goals outside of your sport adds more to your goals? How?

O We can only give away what we have inside ourselves. The great thing is that it will never take from us to support others when we have it for ourselves first. What do you see in others? If it is ugliness then love yourself more :)

I AM SO PROUD OF YOU!

FRIDAY DAILY JOURNALING   DATE _____

JOURNALING PROMPTS

O Pick your intentional word or phrase of the day. Think about your week. What can you focus on today that will support your entire week?

_____

O Can you think of situations this week where you were more in your own A Circle?

_____
_____
_____
_____

O How was that helpful for you?

_____
_____
_____
_____

O When you think about your A Circle, can you see how your ability to manage it can be helpful for your goals? What did you learn this week about how you are able to manage your A Circle?

_____
_____
_____
_____

O Think of situations in the past that did not go well. An injury? Maybe you broke down under pressure, or you were worried about what people were thinking of you. Write them down.

_____
_____
_____

MENTAL STRENGTH COACHING JOURNAL   97

O Looking back, do you see that if you would have known these tools and strategies, they would have been helpful? Remember, you did the best you could with what you knew at the time. What strategies could you have used? What could you have had in your A Circle?

O This week, when you look back, name 3 reasons for your success.

O What do you do well? How do you do it well? Remember: nobody does your skills/ sport/game better than you —be confident in that.

O Step back and practice joy. Where do you have the most joy in your life? Do more of that.

SATURDAY DAILY JOURNALING   DATE _____

CELEBRATION DAY!

O Think of 5 situations where you were successful. Write them down.

_____

_____

_____

_____

_____

_____

O Think of 5 things that you accomplished this week. Write them down.

_____

_____

_____

_____

_____

_____

O Where did you build strength this week mentally? Physically?

_____

_____

_____

_____

_____

_____

O What did you learn from this week that can support you to achieve your goals?

_____

_____

_____

_____

_____

_____

○ What went well? What didn't go well? And what can you learn from both?

○ Remember that you are not equal to the result. When you accomplish a goal, it is fantastic —*but you are not equal to it*. Learn from it so you can use that experience and same strategy to build success. Where this week can you use this?

○ Also, you are not equal to the mistake, or what did not go well. Separate yourself from those situations so that you can also learn from them. Can you think of any situation this week where you can practice this? Are you hard on yourself? Do you have high expectations of yourself? That's okay, but neither of those things belong in your A Circle when you are doing your sport. Did you have situations this week where this got in your way?

SUNDAY! DAILY JOURNALING   DATE _____

DREAM DAY!

O Give yourself permission to dream. We need to practice dreaming. It's not a bad thing to desire, or to want things in your life! Putting your best self into your life, sharing your gift to the world, being more of you, is your responsibility and your job. Dreaming only inspires more of you in that way. As you practice putting more of you into your life, you can share that with others; that is inspiring. Where this week were you more of you?

_____

_____

_____

_____

_____

O Regarding your answer above, were people receptive to it or a little bit threatened?

_____

_____

_____

Remember this: I can only see in you what I have in myself. So, if I don't see you in all your brightness, it's not because something is wrong with *you*. It is *my* lack that is the issue. Do not let someone else's inability to see your light dim it. Practice being your light. Practice seeing other's light as well.

_____

_____

_____

_____

_____

_____

_____

PRACTICE THESE 10 MINDSET RULES:

1 Set big, bold, tremendous goals.

2 Be grateful for everything you have today, and everything you don't have yet.

3 Be 100% accountable for your life. It doesn't mean that everything is your fault, but taking 100% responsibility for it moves you forward with strength.

4 Be thankful – for everything that went well and for everything that didn't go well.

5 Act, speak, think, and perform from the perspective of your Goal Beyond The Goal®.

6 Replace every negative thought with positive thought.

7 Add enthusiasm, energy and certainty to everything in your life!

8 Disregard disempowering actions and language.

9 There are no problems, only opportunities.

10 Bring the data, not the drama!

MONTH _____ 20 _____

MONDAY	TUESDAY	WEDNESDAY	THURSDAY

CONNECT who you are **TO** what you do.
Live in **YOUR POTENTIAL** one day at a time.

© Stacey Herman Goodrich

FRIDAY	SATURDAY	SUNDAY

week 1

MONDAY DAILY JOURNALING   DATE _____

MENTAL MINDSET FOR THE WEEK

Are you achieving your goals? Make sure you set more goals to keep you continually moving forward!

JOURNALING PROMPTS

O Pick an intentional word or phrase of the day that is directly related to your goals. What do you want?

_____

O Think about moving forward. What do you want to have in your A Circle? How will that support you? Today, practice putting more of *you* into your A Circle to move toward your goals.

_____
_____
_____
_____
_____
_____

O Think about what went well and what did not go well in the past. What strategies were you using in those situations? What was in your A Circle?

_____
_____
_____
_____
_____
_____

O How have your strategies evolved in the past three months? What are you more aware of? How have you been more accepting of yourself in your situation(s)?

O What goals have you achieved in the last three months? What strategies did you use to support those goals?

O What do you want to achieve in the next three months?

O What has been in your way of achieving your goals in the past? What is something that you don't want people to know about you? What limiting beliefs do you have about yourself, or your life, or your situation(s)?

TUESDAY DAILY JOURNALING   DATE _____

JOURNALING PROMPTS

O Pick your intentional word or phrase of the day. Again, connect it directly to
your goals.

_____

O How did yesterday's intentional word or phrase of the day support your goals?
How can you support your goals more intentionally?

_____
_____
_____
_____
_____

O What is your goal beyond the goal? Where do you want to be 3 years down
the road?

_____
_____
_____
_____
_____

O What is your goal for the next 3 months? What strategies do you use to support
yourself in achieving your goals during these next 3 months?

_____
_____
_____
_____

MENTAL STRENGTH COACHING JOURNAL   107

O What do you do well? What do people say you do well? What are you good at in
your sport and outside of your sport?

_____

_____

_____

_____

O Think of a situation where something went well. Go into that experience... and
now step out of it. How were you doing that particular thing well? Was it something you saw? Something you felt? Something you said to yourself? Something
you heard? Or a combination?

_____

_____

_____

_____

O This is your strategy for success. Can you use this more often? Where?

_____

_____

_____

_____

O Can you see how you can use this strategy to achieve your goals in the next 3
months? In the next 3 years? How could you have used it this past week?

_____

_____

_____

_____

O What inspired you today?

_____

_____

_____

_____

WEDNESDAY DAILY JOURNALING DATE _____

JOURNALING PROMPTS

O Pick your intentional word or phrase of the day.

_____

O How has the intentional word of the day changed how you live your life?

_____

_____

O Do you like to see your way through your skills/plays/sport? Or feel your way through, think your way through, talk your way through, or a combination?

_____

_____

_____

O Think of a time when you were successful. What strategy were you using? What was in your A Circle?

_____

_____

_____

O Can you practice using this strategy moving forward? In what past situations could you have used this strategy? With coaches? Teammates?

_____

_____

_____

O Really dig down deep to think about what you do well. What gifts do you have that you can become more aware of? I want you to think about where things went really well in the past. How did you contribute to that?

_____

_____

_____

MENTAL STRENGTH COACHING JOURNAL   109

O I am so proud of you. Get comfortable in your success. Know that you always have more to grow and do. BUT, get comfortable in it! We do not have to struggle to be more successful. Where in the past did you sabotage your success or yourself?

O Now, think about how you could have taken care of yourself better in those situations. Could you have gotten stronger without the injury? Could you have been better without struggling for the entire season?

O Do you seek support from outside of yourself or inside of yourself? What works best for you? Do THAT more often. What ever works for you is great. Understanding what you need is what you can practice more.

O Think about your situation. What are some great things about your situation (coaches...team...parents...club...school) that can support you to achieve your goals?

O Outside of your sport —what do you love?

THURSDAY DAILY JOURNALING   DATE _____

JOURNALING PROMPTS

O   What is your intentional word of the day? Pick one that directly connects you to your gift!

_____

O   Remember that you have a "present self "and a "goal self." Practice stepping out of your "present self" and stepping into your "goal self " more often. Add your ability to share your gift with the world more often. What do you do well and how do you do it well? How can you explore ways to do and be more of that??

_____

_____

_____

_____

O   Do you have situations where your A Circle gets crowded with negative thoughts, or negative energy, or negative people? Are you having trouble kicking them out? If you are struggling with negative things in your A Circle, how can you replace them? Do you want to?

_____

_____

_____

_____

O   For example, if you have fear/anxiety/worry in your A Circle, it is only there to help you pay attention, to think about what you want to be doing, or to remind yourself to focus on what you are doing physically. Practice thanking — yes thanking — that energy so you can use it to your advantage. Practice thanking _old_ situations as well. What could you have done to support yourself better in the past?

_____

_____

_____

_____

O Think of some goals outside of your sport that you want to achieve. List them.

O Can you see how adding more of yourself to your goals outside of your sport adds more to your goals? How?

O We can only give away what we have inside ourselves. The great thing is that it will never take from us to support others when we have it for ourselves first. What do you see in others? If it is ugliness then love yourself more :)

I AM SO PROUD OF YOU!

FRIDAY DAILY JOURNALING   DATE _____

JOURNALING PROMPTS

O Pick your intentional word or phrase of the day. Think about your week. What can you focus on today that will support your entire week?

_____

O Can you think of situations this week where you were more in your own A Circle?

_____
_____
_____
_____

O How was that helpful for you?

_____
_____
_____
_____

O When you think about your A Circle, can you see how your ability to manage it can be helpful for your goals? What did you learn this week about how you are able to manage your A Circle?

_____
_____
_____
_____

O Think of situations in the past that did not go well. An injury? Maybe you broke down under pressure, or you were worried about what people were thinking of you. Write them down.

_____
_____
_____

O Looking back, do you see that if you would have known these tools and strategies, they would have been helpful? Remember, you did the best you could with what you knew at the time. What strategies could you have used? What could you have had in your A Circle?

_____

_____

_____

_____

_____

O This week, when you look back, name 3 reasons for your success.

_____

_____

_____

_____

_____

_____

O What do you do well? How do you do it well? Remember: nobody does your skills/ sport/game better than you —be confident in that.

_____

_____

_____

_____

_____

_____

O Step back and practice joy. Where do you have the most joy in your life? Do more of that.

_____

_____

_____

_____

_____

_____

SATURDAY DAILY JOURNALING   DATE _____

CELEBRATION DAY!

O Think of 5 situations where you were successful. Write them down.

_____

_____

_____

_____

_____

_____

O Think of 5 things that you accomplished this week. Write them down.

_____

_____

_____

_____

_____

_____

O Where did you build strength this week mentally? Physically?

_____

_____

_____

_____

_____

O What did you learn from this week that can support you to achieve your goals?

_____

_____

_____

_____

_____

○ What went well? What didn't go well? And what can you learn from both?

○ Remember that you are not equal to the result. When you accomplish a goal, it is fantastic —*but you are not equal to it.* Learn from it so you can use that experience and same strategy to build success. Where this week can you use this?

○ Also, you are not equal to the mistake, or what did not go well. Separate yourself from those situations so that you can also learn from them. Can you think of any situation this week where you can practice this? Are you hard on yourself? Do you have high expectations of yourself? That's okay, but neither of those things belong in your A Circle when you are doing your sport. Did you have situations this week where this got in your way?

SUNDAY! DAILY JOURNALING   DATE _____

DREAM DAY!

O Give yourself permission to dream. We need to practice dreaming. It's not a bad thing to desire, or to want things in your life! Putting your best self into your life, sharing your gift to the world, being more of you, is your responsibility and your job. Dreaming only inspires more of you in that way. As you practice putting more of you into your life, you can share that with others; that is inspiring. Where this week were you more of you?

_____

_____

_____

_____

_____

O Regarding your answer above, were people receptive to it or a little bit threatened?

_____

_____

_____

Remember this: I can only see in you what I have in myself. So, if I don't see you in all your brightness, it's not because something is wrong with *you*. It is *my* lack that is the issue. Do not let someone else's inability to see your light dim it. Practice being your light. Practice seeing other's light as well.

_____

_____

_____

_____

_____

_____

_____

PRACTICE THESE 10 MINDSET RULES:

1 Set big, bold, tremendous goals.

2 Be grateful for everything you have today, and everything you don't have yet.

3 Be 100% accountable for your life. It doesn't mean that everything is your fault, but taking 100% responsibility for it moves you forward with strength.

4 Be thankful – for everything that went well and for everything that didn't go well.

5 Act, speak, think, and perform from the perspective of your Goal Beyond The Goal®.

6 Replace every negative thought with positive thought.

7 Add enthusiasm, energy and certainty to everything in your life!

8 Disregard disempowering actions and language.

9 There are no problems, only opportunities.

10 Bring the data, not the drama!

week 2
MONDAY DAILY JOURNALING   DATE _____

MENTAL MINDSET FOR THE WEEK

Where in the past were you confident? Go back into that experience. How were you doing it? Was it something you felt? Something you heard? Something you saw? Something you said to yourself? A combination? Practice that strategy moving forward to become more confident.

JOURNALING PROMPTS

O Pick an intentional word or phrase of the day that is directly related to your goals. What do you want?

_____

O Think about moving forward. What do you want to have in your A Circle? How will that support you? Today, practice putting more of *you* into your A Circle to move toward your goals.

_____
_____
_____
_____
_____
_____

O Think about what went well and what did not go well in the past. What strategies were you using in those situations? What was in your A Circle?

_____
_____
_____
_____
_____
_____

O How have your strategies evolved in the past three months? What are you more aware of? How have you been more accepting of yourself in your situation(s)?

O What goals have you achieved in the last three months? What strategies did you use to support those goals?

O What do you want to achieve in the next three months?

O What has been in your way of achieving your goals in the past? What is something that you don't want people to know about you? What limiting beliefs do you have about yourself, or your life, or your situation(s)?

TUESDAY DAILY JOURNALING   DATE _____

JOURNALING PROMPTS

O Pick your intentional word or phrase of the day. Again, connect it directly to your goals.

_____

O How did yesterday's intentional word or phrase of the day support your goals? How can you support your goals more intentionally?

_____
_____
_____
_____

O What is your goal beyond the goal? Where do you want to be 3 years down the road?

_____
_____
_____
_____

O What is your goal for the next 3 months? What strategies do you use to support yourself in achieving your goals during these next 3 months?

_____
_____
_____

MENTAL STRENGTH COACHING JOURNAL   121

O What do you do well? What do people say you do well? What are you good at in your sport and outside of your sport?

O Think of a situation where something went well. Go into that experience... and now step out of it. How were you doing that particular thing well? Was it something you saw? Something you felt? Something you said to yourself? Something you heard? Or a combination?

O This is your strategy for success. Can you use this more often? Where?

O Can you see how you can use this strategy to achieve your goals in the next 3 months? In the next 3 years? How could you have used it this past week?

O What inspired you today?

WEDNESDAY DAILY JOURNALING DATE _____

JOURNALING PROMPTS

O Pick your intentional word or phrase of the day.

_____

O How has the intentional word of the day changed how you live your life?

_____

_____

O Do you like to see your way through your skills/plays/sport? Or feel your way through, think your way through, talk your way through, or a combination?

_____

_____

_____

O Think of a time when you were successful. What strategy were you using? What was in your A Circle?

_____

_____

_____

O Can you practice using this strategy moving forward? In what past situations could you have used this strategy? With coaches? Teammates?

_____

_____

_____

O Really dig down deep to think about what you do well. What gifts do you have that you can become more aware of? I want you to think about where things went really well in the past. How did you contribute to that?

_____

_____

_____

O I am so proud of you. Get comfortable in your success. Know that you always have more to grow and do. BUT, get comfortable in it! We do not have to struggle to be more successful. Where in the past did you sabotage your success or yourself?

_____

_____

_____

_____

O Now, think about how you could have taken care of yourself better in those situations. Could you have gotten stronger without the injury? Could you have been better without struggling for the entire season?

_____

_____

_____

O Do you seek support from outside of yourself or inside of yourself? What works best for you? Do THAT more often. What ever works for you is great. Understanding what you need is what you can practice more.

_____

_____

_____

O Think about your situation. What are some great things about your situation (coaches...team...parents...club...school) that can support you to achieve your goals?

_____

_____

_____

O Outside of your sport —what do you love?

_____

_____

_____

_____

THURSDAY DAILY JOURNALING   DATE _____

JOURNALING PROMPTS

O What is your intentional word of the day? Pick one that directly connects you to your gift!

_____

O Remember that you have a "present self "and a "goal self." Practice stepping out of your "present self" and stepping into your "goal self " more often. Add your ability to share your gift with the world more often. What do you do well and how do you do it well? How can you explore ways to do and be more of that??

_____
_____
_____
_____

O Do you have situations where your A Circle gets crowded with negative thoughts, or negative energy, or negative people? Are you having trouble kicking them out? If you are struggling with negative things in your A Circle, how can you replace them? Do you want to?

_____
_____
_____
_____

O For example, if you have fear/anxiety/worry in your A Circle, it is only there to help you pay attention, to think about what you want to be doing, or to remind yourself to focus on what you are doing physically. Practice thanking — yes thanking — that energy so you can use it to your advantage. Practice thanking *old* situations as well. What could you have done to support yourself better in the past?

_____
_____
_____
_____

O Think of some goals outside of your sport that you want to achieve. List them.

O Can you see how adding more of yourself to your goals outside of your sport adds more to your goals? How?

O We can only give away what we have inside ourselves. The great thing is that it will never take from us to support others when we have it for ourselves first. What do you see in others? If it is ugliness then love yourself more :)

I AM SO PROUD OF YOU!

FRIDAY DAILY JOURNALING   DATE _____

JOURNALING PROMPTS

O Pick your intentional word or phrase of the day. Think about your week. What can you focus on today that will support your entire week?

_____

O Can you think of situations this week where you were more in your own A Circle?

_____
_____
_____
_____

O How was that helpful for you?

_____
_____
_____
_____

O When you think about your A Circle, can you see how your ability to manage it can be helpful for your goals? What did you learn this week about how you are able to manage your A Circle?

_____
_____
_____
_____

O Think of situations in the past that did not go well. An injury? Maybe you broke down under pressure, or you were worried about what people were thinking of you. Write them down.

_____
_____
_____
_____

○ Looking back, do you see that if you would have known these tools and strategies, they would have been helpful? Remember, you did the best you could with what you knew at the time. What strategies could you have used? What could you have had in your A Circle?

○ This week, when you look back, name 3 reasons for your success.

○ What do you do well? How do you do it well? Remember: nobody does your skills/sport/game better than you —be confident in that.

○ Step back and practice joy. Where do you have the most joy in your life? Do more of that.

SATURDAY DAILY JOURNALING   DATE _____

CELEBRATION DAY!

O Think of 5 situations where you were successful. Write them down.

_____

_____

_____

_____

_____

_____

O Think of 5 things that you accomplished this week. Write them down.

_____

_____

_____

_____

_____

_____

O Where did you build strength this week mentally? Physically?

_____

_____

_____

_____

_____

_____

O What did you learn from this week that can support you to achieve your goals?

_____

_____

_____

_____

_____

_____

○ What went well? What didn't go well? And what can you learn from both?

○ Remember that you are not equal to the result. When you accomplish a goal, it is fantastic —*but you are not equal to it.* Learn from it so you can use that experience and same strategy to build success. Where this week can you use this?

○ Also, you are not equal to the mistake, or what did not go well. Separate yourself from those situations so that you can also learn from them. Can you think of any situation this week where you can practice this? Are you hard on yourself? Do you have high expectations of yourself? That's okay, but neither of those things belong in your A Circle when you are doing your sport. Did you have situations this week where this got in your way?

SUNDAY! DAILY JOURNALING   DATE _____

DREAM DAY!

○ Give yourself permission to dream. We need to practice dreaming. It's not a bad thing to desire, or to want things in your life! Putting your best self into your life, sharing your gift to the world, being more of you, is your responsibility and your job. Dreaming only inspires more of you in that way. As you practice putting more of you into your life, you can share that with others; that is inspiring. Where this week were you more of you?

_____

_____

_____

_____

_____

○ Regarding your answer above, were people receptive to it or a little bit threatened?

_____

_____

_____

Remember this: I can only see in you what I have in myself. So, if I don't see you in all your brightness, it's not because something is wrong with *you*. It is *my* lack that is the issue. Do not let someone else's inability to see your light dim it. Practice being your light. Practice seeing other's light as well.

_____

_____

_____

_____

_____

_____

_____

PRACTICE THESE 10 MINDSET RULES:

1 Set big, bold, tremendous goals.

2 Be grateful for everything you have today, and everything you don't have yet.

3 Be 100% accountable for your life. It doesn't mean that everything is your fault, but taking 100% responsibility for it moves you forward with strength.

4 Be thankful – for everything that went well and for everything that didn't go well.

5 Act, speak, think, and perform from the perspective of your Goal Beyond The Goal®.

6 Replace every negative thought with positive thought.

7 Add enthusiasm, energy and certainty to everything in your life!

8 Disregard disempowering actions and language.

9 There are no problems, only opportunities.

10 Bring the data, not the drama!

week 3

MONDAY DAILY JOURNALING   DATE _____

MENTAL MINDSET FOR THE WEEK

Step back and think about where you were mentally before you started this journal series. How have you changed? How has your mindset been helpful? Do you see how you can continue to achieve your goals moving forward?

JOURNALING PROMPTS

O Pick an intentional word or phrase of the day that is directly related to your goals. What do you want?

_____

O Think about moving forward. What do you want to have in your A Circle? How will that support you? Today, practice putting more of *you* into your A Circle to move toward your goals.

_____
_____
_____
_____
_____
_____
_____

O Think about what went well and what did not go well in the past. What strategies were you using in those situations? What was in your A Circle?

_____
_____
_____
_____
_____
_____

O How have your strategies evolved in the past three months? What are you more aware of? How have you been more accepting of yourself in your situation(s)?

O What goals have you achieved in the last three months? What strategies did you use to support those goals?

O What do you want to achieve in the next three months?

O What has been in your way of achieving your goals in the past? What is something that you don't want people to know about you? What limiting beliefs do you have about yourself, or your life, or your situation(s)?

TUESDAY DAILY JOURNALING   DATE _____

JOURNALING PROMPTS

O Pick your intentional word or phrase of the day. Again, connect it directly to
your goals.

_____

O How did yesterday's intentional word or phrase of the day support your goals?
How can you support your goals more intentionally?

_____
_____
_____
_____
_____

O What is your goal beyond the goal? Where do you want to be 3 years down
the road?

_____
_____
_____
_____
_____

O What is your goal for the next 3 months? What strategies do you use to support
yourself in achieving your goals during these next 3 months?

_____
_____
_____
_____

O What do you do well? What do people say you do well? What are you good at in your sport and outside of your sport?

O Think of a situation where something went well. Go into that experience... and now step out of it. How were you doing that particular thing well? Was it something you saw? Something you felt? Something you said to yourself? Something you heard? Or a combination?

O This is your strategy for success. Can you use this more often? Where?

O Can you see how you can use this strategy to achieve your goals in the next 3 months? In the next 3 years? How could you have used it this past week?

O What inspired you today?

WEDNESDAY DAILY JOURNALING   DATE _____

JOURNALING PROMPTS

O Pick your intentional word or phrase of the day.

_____

O How has the intentional word of the day changed how you live your life?

_____
_____

O Do you like to see your way through your skills/plays/sport? Or feel your way
through, think your way through, talk your way through, or a combination?

_____
_____
_____

O Think of a time when you were successful. What strategy were you using? What
was in your A Circle?

_____
_____
_____

O Can you practice using this strategy moving forward? In what past situations could
you have used this strategy? With coaches? Teammates?

_____
_____
_____

O Really dig down deep to think about what you do well. What gifts do you have that
you can become more aware of? I want you to think about where things went really
well in the past. How did you contribute to that?

_____
_____
_____

○ I am so proud of you. Get comfortable in your success. Know that you always have more to grow and do. BUT, get comfortable in it! We do not have to struggle to be more successful. Where in the past did you sabotage your success or yourself?

○ Now, think about how you could have taken care of yourself better in those situations. Could you have gotten stronger without the injury? Could you have been better without struggling for the entire season?

○ Do you seek support from outside of yourself or inside of yourself? What works best for you? Do THAT more often. What ever works for you is great. Understanding what you need is what you can practice more.

○ Think about your situation. What are some great things about your situation (coaches...team...parents...club...school) that can support you to achieve your goals?

○ Outside of your sport —what do you love?

THURSDAY DAILY JOURNALING　　DATE _____

JOURNALING PROMPTS

O What is your intentional word of the day? Pick one that directly connects you to your gift!

_____

O Remember that you have a "present self "and a "goal self." Practice stepping out of your "present self" and stepping into your "goal self " more often. Add your ability to share your gift with the world more often. What do you do well and how do you do it well? How can you explore ways to do and be more of that??

_____
_____
_____
_____

O Do you have situations where your A Circle gets crowded with negative thoughts, or negative energy, or negative people? Are you having trouble kicking them out? If you are struggling with negative things in your A Circle, how can you replace them? Do you want to?

_____
_____
_____
_____

O For example, if you have fear/anxiety/worry in your A Circle, it is only there to help you pay attention, to think about what you want to be doing, or to remind yourself to focus on what you are doing physically. Practice thanking — yes thanking — that energy so you can use it to your advantage. Practice thanking *old* situations as well. What could you have done to support yourself better in the past?

_____
_____
_____
_____

O Think of some goals outside of your sport that you want to achieve. List them.

O Can you see how adding more of yourself to your goals outside of your sport adds more to your goals? How?

O We can only give away what we have inside ourselves. The great thing is that it will never take from us to support others when we have it for ourselves first. What do you see in others? If it is ugliness then love yourself more :)

I AM SO PROUD OF YOU!

FRIDAY DAILY JOURNALING   DATE _____

JOURNALING PROMPTS

O Pick your intentional word or phrase of the day. Think about your week. What can you focus on today that will support your entire week?

_____

O Can you think of situations this week where you were more in your own A Circle?

_____
_____
_____
_____

O How was that helpful for you?

_____
_____
_____
_____

O When you think about your A Circle, can you see how your ability to manage it can be helpful for your goals? What did you learn this week about how you are able to manage your A Circle?

_____
_____
_____
_____

O Think of situations in the past that did not go well. An injury? Maybe you broke down under pressure, or you were worried about what people were thinking of you. Write them down.

_____
_____
_____
_____

MENTAL STRENGTH COACHING JOURNAL   141

O Looking back, do you see that if you would have known these tools and strategies, they would have been helpful? Remember, you did the best you could with what you knew at the time. What strategies could you have used? What could you have had in your A Circle?

O This week, when you look back, name 3 reasons for your success.

O What do you do well? How do you do it well? Remember: nobody does your skills/sport/game better than you —be confident in that.

O Step back and practice joy. Where do you have the most joy in your life? Do more of that.

SATURDAY DAILY JOURNALING   DATE _____

CELEBRATION DAY!

O Think of 5 situations where you were successful. Write them down.

_____

_____

_____

_____

_____

_____

O Think of 5 things that you accomplished this week. Write them down.

_____

_____

_____

_____

_____

_____

O Where did you build strength this week mentally? Physically?

_____

_____

_____

_____

_____

_____

O What did you learn from this week that can support you to achieve your goals?

_____

_____

_____

_____

_____

_____

O What went well? What didn't go well? And what can you learn from both?

O Remember that you are not equal to the result. When you accomplish a goal, it is fantastic —*but you are not equal to it.* Learn from it so you can use that experience and same strategy to build success. Where this week can you use this?

O Also, you are not equal to the mistake, or what did not go well. Separate yourself from those situations so that you can also learn from them. Can you think of any situation this week where you can practice this? Are you hard on yourself? Do you have high expectations of yourself? That's okay, but neither of those things belong in your A Circle when you are doing your sport. Did you have situations this week where this got in your way?

SUNDAY! DAILY JOURNALING DATE _____

DREAM DAY!

O Give yourself permission to dream. We need to practice dreaming. It's not a bad thing to desire, or to want things in your life! Putting your best self into your life, sharing your gift to the world, being more of you, is your responsibility and your job. Dreaming only inspires more of you in that way. As you practice putting more of you into your life, you can share that with others; that is inspiring. Where this week were you more of you?

_____

_____

_____

_____

_____

O Regarding your answer above, were people receptive to it or a little bit threatened?

_____

_____

Remember this: I can only see in you what I have in myself. So, if I don't see you in all your brightness, it's not because something is wrong with *you*. It is *my* lack that is the issue. Do not let someone else's inability to see your light dim it. Practice being your light. Practice seeing other's light as well.

_____

_____

_____

_____

_____

_____

PRACTICE THESE 10 MINDSET RULES:

1 Set big, bold, tremendous goals.

2 Be grateful for everything you have today, and everything you don't have yet.

3 Be 100% accountable for your life. It doesn't mean that everything is your fault, but taking 100% responsibility for it moves you forward with strength.

4 Be thankful – for everything that went well and for everything that didn't go well.

5 Act, speak, think, and perform from the perspective of your Goal Beyond The Goal®.

6 Replace every negative thought with positive thought.

7 Add enthusiasm, energy and certainty to everything in your life!

8 Disregard disempowering actions and language.

9 There are no problems, only opportunities.

10 Bring the data, not the drama!

week 4

MONDAY DAILY JOURNALING   DATE _____

MENTAL MINDSET FOR THE WEEK

You can do anything you set your mind to!

JOURNALING PROMPTS

O Pick an intentional word or phrase of the day that is directly related to your goals. What do you want?

_____

O Think about moving forward. What do you want to have in your A Circle? How will that support you? Today, practice putting more of *you* into your A Circle to move toward your goals.

_____
_____
_____
_____
_____
_____

O Think about what went well and what did not go well in the past. What strategies were you using in those situations? What was in your A Circle?

_____
_____
_____
_____
_____
_____
_____

O How have your strategies evolved in the past three months? What are you more aware of? How have you been more accepting of yourself in your situation(s)?

O What goals have you achieved in the last three months? What strategies did you use to support those goals?

O What do you want to achieve in the next three months?

O What has been in your way of achieving your goals in the past? What is something that you don't want people to know about you? What limiting beliefs do you have about yourself, or your life, or your situation(s)?

TUESDAY DAILY JOURNALING   DATE _____

JOURNALING PROMPTS

O Pick your intentional word or phrase of the day. Again, connect it directly to
your goals.

_____

O How did yesterday's intentional word or phrase of the day support your goals?
How can you support your goals more intentionally?

_____
_____
_____
_____
_____

O What is your goal beyond the goal? Where do you want to be 3 years down
the road?

_____
_____
_____
_____
_____

O What is your goal for the next 3 months? What strategies do you use to support
yourself in achieving your goals during these next 3 months?

_____
_____
_____
_____

MENTAL STRENGTH COACHING JOURNAL   149

○ What do you do well? What do people say you do well? What are you good at in your sport and outside of your sport?

○ Think of a situation where something went well. Go into that experience... and now step out of it. How were you doing that particular thing well? Was it something you saw? Something you felt? Something you said to yourself? Something you heard? Or a combination?

○ This is your strategy for success. Can you use this more often? Where?

○ Can you see how you can use this strategy to achieve your goals in the next 3 months? In the next 3 years? How could you have used it this past week?

○ What inspired you today?

WEDNESDAY DAILY JOURNALING   DATE _____

JOURNALING PROMPTS

O Pick your intentional word or phrase of the day.

_____

O How has the intentional word of the day changed how you live your life?

_____

_____

O Do you like to see your way through your skills/plays/sport? Or feel your way
   through, think your way through, talk your way through, or a combination?

_____

_____

_____

O Think of a time when you were successful. What strategy were you using? What
   was in your A Circle?

_____

_____

_____

O Can you practice using this strategy moving forward? In what past situations could
   you have used this strategy? With coaches? Teammates?

_____

_____

_____

O Really dig down deep to think about what you do well. What gifts do you have that
   you can become more aware of? I want you to think about where things went really
   well in the past. How did you contribute to that?

_____

_____

_____

O I am so proud of you. Get comfortable in your success. Know that you always have more to grow and do. BUT, get comfortable in it! We do not have to struggle to be more successful. Where in the past did you sabotage your success or yourself?

O Now, think about how you could have taken care of yourself better in those situations. Could you have gotten stronger without the injury? Could you have been better without struggling for the entire season?

O Do you seek support from outside of yourself or inside of yourself? What works best for you? Do THAT more often. What ever works for you is great. Understanding what you need is what you can practice more.

O Think about your situation. What are some great things about your situation (coaches...team...parents...club...school) that can support you to achieve your goals?

O Outside of your sport —what do you love?

THURSDAY DAILY JOURNALING   DATE _____

JOURNALING PROMPTS

○ What is your intentional word of the day? Pick one that directly connects you to your gift!

_____

○ Remember that you have a "present self "and a "goal self." Practice stepping out of your "present self" and stepping into your "goal self " more often. Add your ability to share your gift with the world more often. What do you do well and how do you do it well? How can you explore ways to do and be more of that??

_____
_____
_____
_____

○ Do you have situations where your A Circle gets crowded with negative thoughts, or negative energy, or negative people? Are you having trouble kicking them out? If you are struggling with negative things in your A Circle, how can you replace them? Do you want to?

_____
_____
_____
_____

○ For example, if you have fear/anxiety/worry in your A Circle, it is only there to help you pay attention, to think about what you want to be doing, or to remind yourself to focus on what you are doing physically. Practice thanking — yes thanking — that energy so you can use it to your advantage. Practice thanking *old* situations as well. What could you have done to support yourself better in the past?

_____
_____
_____
_____

O Think of some goals outside of your sport that you want to achieve. List them.

O Can you see how adding more of yourself to your goals outside of your sport adds more to your goals? How?

O We can only give away what we have inside ourselves. The great thing is that it will never take from us to support others when we have it for ourselves first. What do you see in others? If it is ugliness then love yourself more :)

I AM SO PROUD OF YOU!

FRIDAY DAILY JOURNALING DATE _____

JOURNALING PROMPTS

O Pick your intentional word or phrase of the day. Think about your week. What can you focus on today that will support your entire week?

_____

O Can you think of situations this week where you were more in your own A Circle?

_____
_____
_____
_____

O How was that helpful for you?

_____
_____
_____
_____

O When you think about your A Circle, can you see how your ability to manage it can be helpful for your goals? What did you learn this week about how you are able to manage your A Circle?

_____
_____
_____
_____

O Think of situations in the past that did not go well. An injury? Maybe you broke down under pressure, or you were worried about what people were thinking of you. Write them down.

_____
_____
_____
_____

O Looking back, do you see that if you would have known these tools and strategies, they would have been helpful? Remember, you did the best you could with what you knew at the time. What strategies could you have used? What could you have had in your A Circle?

_____

_____

_____

_____

_____

O This week, when you look back, name 3 reasons for your success.

_____

_____

_____

_____

_____

O What do you do well? How do you do it well? Remember: nobody does your skills/sport/game better than you —be confident in that.

_____

_____

_____

_____

_____

O Step back and practice joy. Where do you have the most joy in your life? Do more of that.

_____

_____

_____

_____

_____

SATURDAY DAILY JOURNALING   DATE _____

CELEBRATION DAY!

O Think of 5 situations where you were successful. Write them down.

_____

_____

_____

_____

_____

_____

O Think of 5 things that you accomplished this week. Write them down.

_____

_____

_____

_____

_____

_____

O Where did you build strength this week mentally? Physically?

_____

_____

_____

_____

_____

_____

O What did you learn from this week that can support you to achieve your goals?

_____

_____

_____

_____

_____

O What went well? What didn't go well? And what can you learn from both?

O Remember that you are not equal to the result. When you accomplish a goal, it is fantastic —*but you are not equal to it*. Learn from it so you can use that experience and same strategy to build success. Where this week can you use this?

O Also, you are not equal to the mistake, or what did not go well. Separate yourself from those situations so that you can also learn from them. Can you think of any situation this week where you can practice this? Are you hard on yourself? Do you have high expectations of yourself? That's okay, but neither of those things belong in your A Circle when you are doing your sport. Did you have situations this week where this got in your way?

SUNDAY! DAILY JOURNALING   DATE _____

DREAM DAY!

O Give yourself permission to dream. We need to practice dreaming. It's not a bad thing to desire, or to want things in your life! Putting your best self into your life, sharing your gift to the world, being more of you, is your responsibility and your job. Dreaming only inspires more of you in that way. As you practice putting more of you into your life, you can share that with others; that is inspiring. Where this week were you more of you?

_____

_____

_____

_____

_____

O Regarding your answer above, were people receptive to it or a little bit threatened?

_____

_____

_____

Remember this: I can only see in you what I have in myself. So, if I don't see you in all your brightness, it's not because something is wrong with *you*. It is *my* lack that is the issue. Do not let someone else's inability to see your light dim it. Practice being your light. Practice seeing other's light as well.

_____

_____

_____

_____

_____

_____

_____

PRACTICE THESE 10 MINDSET RULES:

1 Set big, bold, tremendous goals.

2 Be grateful for everything you have today, and everything you don't have yet.

3 Be 100% accountable for your life. It doesn't mean that everything is your fault, but taking 100% responsibility for it moves you forward with strength.

4 Be thankful – for everything that went well and for everything that didn't go well.

5 Act, speak, think, and perform from the perspective of your Goal Beyond The Goal®.

6 Replace every negative thought with positive thought.

7 Add enthusiasm, energy and certainty to everything in your life!

8 Disregard disempowering actions and language.

9 There are no problems, only opportunities.

10 Bring the data, not the drama!

week 5

MONDAY DAILY JOURNALING   DATE _____

MENTAL MINDSET FOR THE WEEK

Where last week did you tap into your potential? Practice doing that more often!

JOURNALING PROMPTS

O Pick an intentional word or phrase of the day that is directly related to your goals. What do you want?

_____

O Think about moving forward. What do you want to have in your A Circle? How will that support you? Today, practice putting more of *you* into your A Circle to move toward your goals.

_____
_____
_____
_____
_____
_____

O Think about what went well and what did not go well in the past. What strategies were you using in those situations? What was in your A Circle?

_____
_____
_____
_____
_____
_____

O How have your strategies evolved in the past three months? What are you more aware of? How have you been more accepting of yourself in your situation(s)?

O What goals have you achieved in the last three months? What strategies did you use to support those goals?

O What do you want to achieve in the next three months?

O What has been in your way of achieving your goals in the past? What is something that you don't want people to know about you? What limiting beliefs do you have about yourself, or your life, or your situation(s)?

TUESDAY DAILY JOURNALING   DATE _____

JOURNALING PROMPTS

O Pick your intentional word or phrase of the day. Again, connect it directly to
your goals.

_____

O How did yesterday's intentional word or phrase of the day support your goals?
How can you support your goals more intentionally?

_____
_____
_____
_____
_____

O What is your goal beyond the goal? Where do you want to be 3 years down
the road?

_____
_____
_____
_____
_____

O What is your goal for the next 3 months? What strategies do you use to support
yourself in achieving your goals during these next 3 months?

_____
_____
_____
_____

MENTAL STRENGTH COACHING JOURNAL   163

O What do you do well? What do people say you do well? What are you good at in
   your sport and outside of your sport?

_____

_____

_____

_____

O Think of a situation where something went well. Go into that experience... and
   now step out of it. How were you doing that particular thing well? Was it something you saw? Something you felt? Something you said to yourself? Something
   you heard? Or a combination?

_____

_____

_____

_____

O This is your strategy for success. Can you use this more often? Where?

_____

_____

_____

_____

O Can you see how you can use this strategy to achieve your goals in the next 3
   months? In the next 3 years? How could you have used it this past week?

_____

_____

_____

_____

O What inspired you today?

_____

_____

_____

_____

WEDNESDAY DAILY JOURNALING   DATE _____

JOURNALING PROMPTS

O Pick your intentional word or phrase of the day.

_____

O How has the intentional word of the day changed how you live your life?

_____

_____

O Do you like to see your way through your skills/plays/sport? Or feel your way
   through, think your way through, talk your way through, or a combination?

_____

_____

_____

O Think of a time when you were successful. What strategy were you using? What
   was in your A Circle?

_____

_____

_____

O Can you practice using this strategy moving forward? In what past situations could
   you have used this strategy? With coaches? Teammates?

_____

_____

_____

O Really dig down deep to think about what you do well. What gifts do you have that
   you can become more aware of? I want you to think about where things went really
   well in the past. How did you contribute to that?

_____

_____

_____

O I am so proud of you. Get comfortable in your success. Know that you always have more to grow and do. BUT, get comfortable in it! We do not have to struggle to be more successful. Where in the past did you sabotage your success or yourself?

_____

_____

_____

_____

O Now, think about how you could have taken care of yourself better in those situations. Could you have gotten stronger without the injury? Could you have been better without struggling for the entire season?

_____

_____

_____

O Do you seek support from outside of yourself or inside of yourself? What works best for you? Do THAT more often. What ever works for you is great. Understanding what you need is what you can practice more.

_____

_____

_____

O Think about your situation. What are some great things about your situation (coaches...team...parents...club...school) that can support you to achieve your goals?

_____

_____

_____

O Outside of your sport —what do you love?

_____

_____

_____

_____

THURSDAY DAILY JOURNALING   DATE _____

JOURNALING PROMPTS

○ What is your intentional word of the day? Pick one that directly connects you to your gift!

_____

○ Remember that you have a "present self "and a "goal self." Practice stepping out of your "present self" and stepping into your "goal self " more often. Add your ability to share your gift with the world more often. What do you do well and how do you do it well? How can you explore ways to do and be more of that??

_____
_____
_____
_____

○ Do you have situations where your A Circle gets crowded with negative thoughts, or negative energy, or negative people? Are you having trouble kicking them out? If you are struggling with negative things in your A Circle, how can you replace them? Do you want to?

_____
_____
_____
_____

○ For example, if you have fear/anxiety/worry in your A Circle, it is only there to help you pay attention, to think about what you want to be doing, or to remind yourself to focus on what you are doing physically. Practice thanking — yes thanking — that energy so you can use it to your advantage. Practice thanking *old* situations as well. What could you have done to support yourself better in the past?

_____
_____
_____
_____

- Think of some goals outside of your sport that you want to achieve. List them.

- Can you see how adding more of yourself to your goals outside of your sport adds more to your goals? How?

- We can only give away what we have inside ourselves. The great thing is that it will never take from us to support others when we have it for ourselves first. What do you see in others? If it is ugliness then love yourself more :)

I AM SO PROUD OF YOU!

FRIDAY DAILY JOURNALING   DATE _____

JOURNALING PROMPTS

○ Pick your intentional word or phrase of the day. Think about your week. What can you focus on today that will support your entire week?

_____

○ Can you think of situations this week where you were more in your own A Circle?

_____
_____
_____
_____

○ How was that helpful for you?

_____
_____
_____
_____

○ When you think about your A Circle, can you see how your ability to manage it can be helpful for your goals? What did you learn this week about how you are able to manage your A Circle?

_____
_____
_____
_____

○ Think of situations in the past that did not go well. An injury? Maybe you broke down under pressure, or you were worried about what people were thinking of you. Write them down.

_____
_____
_____
_____

O Looking back, do you see that if you would have known these tools and strategies, they would have been helpful? Remember, you did the best you could with what you knew at the time. What strategies could you have used? What could you have had in your A Circle?

O This week, when you look back, name 3 reasons for your success.

O What do you do well? How do you do it well? Remember: nobody does your skills/sport/game better than you —be confident in that.

O Step back and practice joy. Where do you have the most joy in your life? Do more of that.

SATURDAY DAILY JOURNALING   DATE _____

CELEBRATION DAY!

O Think of 5 situations where you were successful. Write them down.

_____
_____
_____
_____
_____
_____

O Think of 5 things that you accomplished this week. Write them down.

_____
_____
_____
_____
_____
_____

O Where did you build strength this week mentally? Physically?

_____
_____
_____
_____
_____
_____

O What did you learn from this week that can support you to achieve your goals?

_____
_____
_____
_____
_____

O What went well? What didn't go well? And what can you learn from both?

O Remember that you are not equal to the result. When you accomplish a goal, it is fantastic —*but you are not equal to it.* Learn from it so you can use that experience and same strategy to build success. Where this week can you use this?

O Also, you are not equal to the mistake, or what did not go well. Separate yourself from those situations so that you can also learn from them. Can you think of any situation this week where you can practice this? Are you hard on yourself? Do you have high expectations of yourself? That's okay, but neither of those things belong in your A Circle when you are doing your sport. Did you have situations this week where this got in your way?

SUNDAY! DAILY JOURNALING   DATE _____

DREAM DAY!

O Give yourself permission to dream. We need to practice dreaming. It's not a bad thing to desire, or to want things in your life! Putting your best self into your life, sharing your gift to the world, being more of you, is your responsibility and your job. Dreaming only inspires more of you in that way. As you practice putting more of you into your life, you can share that with others; that is inspiring. Where this week were you more of you?

_____

_____

_____

_____

_____

O Regarding your answer above, were people receptive to it or a little bit threatened?

_____

_____

_____

Remember this: I can only see in you what I have in myself. So, if I don't see you in all your brightness, it's not because something is wrong with *you*. It is *my* lack that is the issue. Do not let someone else's inability to see your light dim it. Practice being your light. Practice seeing other's light as well.

_____

_____

_____

_____

_____

_____

PRACTICE THESE 10 MINDSET RULES:

1 Set big, bold, tremendous goals.

2 Be grateful for everything you have today, and everything you don't have yet.

3 Be 100% accountable for your life. It doesn't mean that everything is your fault, but taking 100% responsibility for it moves you forward with strength.

4 Be thankful – for everything that went well and for everything that didn't go well.

5 Act, speak, think, and perform from the perspective of your Goal Beyond The Goal®.

6 Replace every negative thought with positive thought.

7 Add enthusiasm, energy and certainty to everything in your life!

8 Disregard disempowering actions and language.

9 There are no problems, only opportunities.

10 Bring the data, not the drama!

MONTH _____ 20 ____

MONDAY	TUESDAY	WEDNESDAY	THURSDAY

CONNECT who you are TO what you do.
Live in YOUR POTENTIAL one day at a time.

© Stacey Herman Goodrich

FRIDAY	SATURDAY	SUNDAY

week 1

MONDAY DAILY JOURNALING   DATE _____

MENTAL MINDSET FOR THE WEEK

Where are you using these strategies in your life outside of the sport? Isn't is great?

JOURNALING PROMPTS

O Pick an intentional word or phrase of the day that is directly related to your goals. What do you want?

_____

O Think about moving forward. What do you want to have in your A Circle? How will that support you? Today, practice putting more of *you* into your A Circle to move toward your goals.

_____
_____
_____
_____
_____
_____

O Think about what went well and what did not go well in the past. What strategies were you using in those situations? What was in your A Circle?

_____
_____
_____
_____
_____

MENTAL STRENGTH COACHING JOURNAL   177

O How have your strategies evolved in the past three months? What are you more
   aware of? How have you been more accepting of yourself in your situation(s)?

O What goals have you achieved in the last three months? What strategies did you
   use to support those goals?

O What do you want to achieve in the next three months?

O What has been in your way of achieving your goals in the past? What is something
   that you don't want people to know about you? What limiting beliefs do you have
   about yourself, or your life, or your situation(s)?

TUESDAY DAILY JOURNALING   DATE _____

JOURNALING PROMPTS

O Pick your intentional word or phrase of the day. Again, connect it directly to your goals.

_____

O How did yesterday's intentional word or phrase of the day support your goals? How can you support your goals more intentionally?

_____

_____

_____

_____

_____

O What is your goal beyond the goal? Where do you want to be 3 years down the road?

_____

_____

_____

_____

_____

O What is your goal for the next 3 months? What strategies do you use to support yourself in achieving your goals during these next 3 months?

_____

_____

_____

_____

MENTAL STRENGTH COACHING JOURNAL   179

O What do you do well? What do people say you do well? What are you good at in
   your sport and outside of your sport?

_____

_____

_____

_____

O Think of a situation where something went well. Go into that experience... and
   now step out of it. How were you doing that particular thing well? Was it something you saw? Something you felt? Something you said to yourself? Something
   you heard? Or a combination?

_____

_____

_____

_____

O This is your strategy for success. Can you use this more often? Where?

_____

_____

_____

_____

O Can you see how you can use this strategy to achieve your goals in the next 3
   months? In the next 3 years? How could you have used it this past week?

_____

_____

_____

_____

O What inspired you today?

_____

_____

_____

_____

WEDNESDAY DAILY JOURNALING   DATE _____

JOURNALING PROMPTS

O Pick your intentional word or phrase of the day.

_____

O How has the intentional word of the day changed how you live your life?

_____

_____

O Do you like to see your way through your skills/plays/sport? Or feel your way through, think your way through, talk your way through, or a combination?

_____

_____

_____

O Think of a time when you were successful. What strategy were you using? What was in your A Circle?

_____

_____

_____

O Can you practice using this strategy moving forward? In what past situations could you have used this strategy? With coaches? Teammates?

_____

_____

_____

O Really dig down deep to think about what you do well. What gifts do you have that you can become more aware of? I want you to think about where things went really well in the past. How did you contribute to that?

_____

_____

_____

- I am so proud of you. Get comfortable in your success. Know that you always have more to grow and do. BUT, get comfortable in it! We do not have to struggle to be more successful. Where in the past did you sabotage your success or yourself?

- Now, think about how you could have taken care of yourself better in those situations. Could you have gotten stronger without the injury? Could you have been better without struggling for the entire season?

- Do you seek support from outside of yourself or inside of yourself? What works best for you? Do THAT more often. What ever works for you is great. Understanding what you need is what you can practice more.

- Think about your situation. What are some great things about your situation (coaches...team...parents...club...school) that can support you to achieve your goals?

- Outside of your sport —what do you love?

THURSDAY DAILY JOURNALING   DATE _____

JOURNALING PROMPTS

○ What is your intentional word of the day? Pick one that directly connects you to your gift!

_____

○ Remember that you have a "present self "and a "goal self." Practice stepping out of your "present self" and stepping into your "goal self " more often. Add your ability to share your gift with the world more often. What do you do well and how do you do it well? How can you explore ways to do and be more of that??

_____
_____
_____
_____

○ Do you have situations where your A Circle gets crowded with negative thoughts, or negative energy, or negative people? Are you having trouble kicking them out? If you are struggling with negative things in your A Circle, how can you replace them? Do you want to?

_____
_____
_____
_____

○ For example, if you have fear/anxiety/worry in your A Circle, it is only there to help you pay attention, to think about what you want to be doing, or to remind yourself to focus on what you are doing physically. Practice thanking — yes thanking — that energy so you can use it to your advantage. Practice thanking *old* situations as well. What could you have done to support yourself better in the past?

_____
_____
_____
_____

MENTAL STRENGTH COACHING JOURNAL   183

O Think of some goals outside of your sport that you want to achieve. List them.

_____

_____

_____

_____

_____

_____

_____

O Can you see how adding more of yourself to your goals outside of your sport adds more to your goals? How?

_____

_____

_____

_____

_____

_____

O We can only give away what we have inside ourselves. The great thing is that it will never take from us to support others when we have it for ourselves first. What do you see in others? If it is ugliness then love yourself more :)

_____

_____

_____

_____

_____

_____

I AM SO PROUD OF YOU!

FRIDAY DAILY JOURNALING   DATE _____

JOURNALING PROMPTS

O Pick your intentional word or phrase of the day. Think about your week. What can you focus on today that will support your entire week?

_____

O Can you think of situations this week where you were more in your own A Circle?

_____

_____

_____

_____

O How was that helpful for you?

_____

_____

_____

_____

O When you think about your A Circle, can you see how your ability to manage it can be helpful for your goals? What did you learn this week about how you are able to manage your A Circle?

_____

_____

_____

_____

O Think of situations in the past that did not go well. An injury? Maybe you broke down under pressure, or you were worried about what people were thinking of you. Write them down.

_____

_____

_____

_____

O Looking back, do you see that if you would have known these tools and strategies, they would have been helpful? Remember, you did the best you could with what you knew at the time. What strategies could you have used? What could you have had in your A Circle?

O This week, when you look back, name 3 reasons for your success.

O What do you do well? How do you do it well? Remember: nobody does your skills/ sport/game better than you —be confident in that.

O Step back and practice joy. Where do you have the most joy in your life? Do more of that.

SATURDAY DAILY JOURNALING   DATE _____

CELEBRATION DAY!

O Think of 5 situations where you were successful. Write them down.

_____

_____

_____

_____

_____

_____

O Think of 5 things that you accomplished this week. Write them down.

_____

_____

_____

_____

_____

_____

O Where did you build strength this week mentally? Physically?

_____

_____

_____

_____

_____

_____

O What did you learn from this week that can support you to achieve your goals?

_____

_____

_____

_____

_____

_____

○ What went well? What didn't go well? And what can you learn from both?

○ Remember that you are not equal to the result. When you accomplish a goal, it is fantastic —*but you are not equal to it.* Learn from it so you can use that experience and same strategy to build success. Where this week can you use this?

○ Also, you are not equal to the mistake, or what did not go well. Separate yourself from those situations so that you can also learn from them. Can you think of any situation this week where you can practice this? Are you hard on yourself? Do you have high expectations of yourself? That's okay, but neither of those things belong in your A Circle when you are doing your sport. Did you have situations this week where this got in your way?

SUNDAY! DAILY JOURNALING   DATE _____

DREAM DAY!

O Give yourself permission to dream. We need to practice dreaming. It's not a bad thing to desire, or to want things in your life! Putting your best self into your life, sharing your gift to the world, being more of you, is your responsibility and your job. Dreaming only inspires more of you in that way. As you practice putting more of you into your life, you can share that with others; that is inspiring. Where this week were you more of you?

_____

_____

_____

_____

_____

O Regarding your answer above, were people receptive to it or a little bit threatened?

_____

_____

_____

Remember this: I can only see in you what I have in myself. So, if I don't see you in all your brightness, it's not because something is wrong with *you*. It is *my* lack that is the issue. Do not let someone else's inability to see your light dim it. Practice being your light. Practice seeing other's light as well.

_____

_____

_____

_____

_____

_____

_____

PRACTICE THESE 10 MINDSET RULES:

1 Set big, bold, tremendous goals.

2 Be grateful for everything you have today, and everything you don't have yet.

3 Be 100% accountable for your life. It doesn't mean that everything is your fault, but taking 100% responsibility for it moves you forward with strength.

4 Be thankful – for everything that went well and for everything that didn't go well.

5 Act, speak, think, and perform from the perspective of your Goal Beyond The Goal®.

6 Replace every negative thought with positive thought.

7 Add enthusiasm, energy and certainty to everything in your life!

8 Disregard disempowering actions and language.

9 There are no problems, only opportunities.

10 Bring the data, not the drama!

week 2

MONDAY DAILY JOURNALING   DATE _____

MENTAL MINDSET FOR THE WEEK

Have you ordered Book 3? www.so-connected.com/books

JOURNALING PROMPTS

O Pick an intentional word or phrase of the day that is directly related to your goals. What do you want?

_____

O Think about moving forward. What do you want to have in your A Circle? How will that support you? Today, practice putting more of *you* into your A Circle to move toward your goals.

_____
_____
_____
_____
_____
_____
_____

O Think about what went well and what did not go well in the past. What strategies were you using in those situations? What was in your A Circle?

_____
_____
_____
_____
_____
_____
_____

MENTAL STRENGTH COACHING JOURNAL   191

O How have your strategies evolved in the past three months? What are you more aware of? How have you been more accepting of yourself in your situation(s)?

_____

_____

_____

_____

_____

_____

O What goals have you achieved in the last three months? What strategies did you use to support those goals?

_____

_____

_____

_____

_____

_____

O What do you want to achieve in the next three months?

_____

_____

_____

_____

_____

_____

O What has been in your way of achieving your goals in the past? What is something that you don't want people to know about you? What limiting beliefs do you have about yourself, or your life, or your situation(s)?

_____

_____

_____

_____

_____

_____

TUESDAY DAILY JOURNALING   DATE _____

JOURNALING PROMPTS

O Pick your intentional word or phrase of the day. Again, connect it directly to your goals.

_____

O How did yesterday's intentional word or phrase of the day support your goals? How can you support your goals more intentionally?

_____
_____
_____
_____
_____

O What is your goal beyond the goal? Where do you want to be 3 years down the road?

_____
_____
_____
_____
_____

O What is your goal for the next 3 months? What strategies do you use to support yourself in achieving your goals during these next 3 months?

_____
_____
_____
_____

O What do you do well? What do people say you do well? What are you good at in your sport and outside of your sport?

O Think of a situation where something went well. Go into that experience... and now step out of it. How were you doing that particular thing well? Was it something you saw? Something you felt? Something you said to yourself? Something you heard? Or a combination?

O This is your strategy for success. Can you use this more often? Where?

O Can you see how you can use this strategy to achieve your goals in the next 3 months? In the next 3 years? How could you have used it this past week?

O What inspired you today?

WEDNESDAY DAILY JOURNALING   DATE _____

JOURNALING PROMPTS

O Pick your intentional word or phrase of the day.

_____

O How has the intentional word of the day changed how you live your life?

_____

_____

O Do you like to see your way through your skills/plays/sport? Or feel your way
   through, think your way through, talk your way through, or a combination?

_____

_____

_____

O Think of a time when you were successful. What strategy were you using? What
   was in your A Circle?

_____

_____

_____

O Can you practice using this strategy moving forward? In what past situations could
   you have used this strategy? With coaches? Teammates?

_____

_____

_____

O Really dig down deep to think about what you do well. What gifts do you have that
   you can become more aware of? I want you to think about where things went really
   well in the past. How did you contribute to that?

_____

_____

_____

MENTAL STRENGTH COACHING JOURNAL   195

○ I am so proud of you. Get comfortable in your success. Know that you always have
more to grow and do. BUT, get comfortable in it! We do not have to struggle to be
more successful. Where in the past did you sabotage your success or yourself?

○ Now, think about how you could have taken care of yourself better in those situations. Could you have gotten stronger without the injury? Could you have been
better without struggling for the entire season?

○ Do you seek support from outside of yourself or inside of yourself? What works
best for you? Do THAT more often. What ever works for you is great. Understanding what you need is what you can practice more.

○ Think about your situation. What are some great things about your situation
(coaches...team...parents...club...school) that can support you to achieve
your goals?

○ Outside of your sport —what do you love?

THURSDAY DAILY JOURNALING   DATE _____

JOURNALING PROMPTS

O What is your intentional word of the day? Pick one that directly connects you to your gift!

_____

O Remember that you have a "present self "and a "goal self." Practice stepping out of your "present self" and stepping into your "goal self " more often. Add your ability to share your gift with the world more often. What do you do well and how do you do it well? How can you explore ways to do and be more of that??

_____
_____
_____
_____

O Do you have situations where your A Circle gets crowded with negative thoughts, or negative energy, or negative people? Are you having trouble kicking them out? If you are struggling with negative things in your A Circle, how can you replace them? Do you want to?

_____
_____
_____
_____

O For example, if you have fear/anxiety/worry in your A Circle, it is only there to help you pay attention, to think about what you want to be doing, or to remind yourself to focus on what you are doing physically. Practice thanking — yes thanking — that energy so you can use it to your advantage. Practice thanking _old_ situations as well. What could you have done to support yourself better in the past?

_____
_____
_____
_____

○ Think of some goals outside of your sport that you want to achieve. List them.

○ Can you see how adding more of yourself to your goals outside of your sport adds more to your goals? How?

○ We can only give away what we have inside ourselves. The great thing is that it will never take from us to support others when we have it for ourselves first. What do you see in others? If it is ugliness then love yourself more :)

I AM SO PROUD OF YOU!

FRIDAY DAILY JOURNALING   DATE _____

JOURNALING PROMPTS

O Pick your intentional word or phrase of the day. Think about your week. What can
you focus on today that will support your entire week?

_____

O Can you think of situations this week where you were more in your own A Circle?

_____
_____
_____
_____

O How was that helpful for you?

_____
_____
_____
_____

O When you think about your A Circle, can you see how your ability to manage it can
be helpful for your goals? What did you learn this week about how you are able to
manage your A Circle?

_____
_____
_____
_____

O Think of situations in the past that did not go well. An injury? Maybe you broke
down under pressure, or you were worried about what people were thinking of
you. Write them down.

_____
_____
_____
_____

O Looking back, do you see that if you would have known these tools and strategies, they would have been helpful? Remember, you did the best you could with what you knew at the time. What strategies could you have used? What could you have had in your A Circle?

O This week, when you look back, name 3 reasons for your success.

O What do you do well? How do you do it well? Remember: nobody does your skills/ sport/game better than you —be confident in that.

O Step back and practice joy. Where do you have the most joy in your life? Do more of that.

SATURDAY DAILY JOURNALING   DATE _____

CELEBRATION DAY!

O Think of 5 situations where you were successful. Write them down.

_____

_____

_____

_____

_____

_____

O Think of 5 things that you accomplished this week. Write them down.

_____

_____

_____

_____

_____

_____

O Where did you build strength this week mentally? Physically?

_____

_____

_____

_____

_____

_____

O What did you learn from this week that can support you to achieve your goals?

_____

_____

_____

_____

_____

_____

○ What went well? What didn't go well? And what can you learn from both?

○ Remember that you are not equal to the result. When you accomplish a goal, it is fantastic —*but you are not equal to it.* Learn from it so you can use that experience and same strategy to build success. Where this week can you use this?

○ Also, you are not equal to the mistake, or what did not go well. Separate yourself from those situations so that you can also learn from them. Can you think of any situation this week where you can practice this? Are you hard on yourself? Do you have high expectations of yourself? That's okay, but neither of those things belong in your A Circle when you are doing your sport. Did you have situations this week where this got in your way?

SUNDAY! DAILY JOURNALING DATE _____

DREAM DAY!

○ Give yourself permission to dream. We need to practice dreaming. It's not a bad thing to desire, or to want things in your life! Putting your best self into your life, sharing your gift to the world, being more of you, is your responsibility and your job. Dreaming only inspires more of you in that way. As you practice putting more of you into your life, you can share that with others; that is inspiring. Where this week were you more of you?

_____

_____

_____

_____

_____

○ Regarding your answer above, were people receptive to it or a little bit threatened?

_____

_____

_____

Remember this: I can only see in you what I have in myself. So, if I don't see you in all your brightness, it's not because something is wrong with *you*. It is *my* lack that is the issue. Do not let someone else's inability to see your light dim it. Practice being your light. Practice seeing other's light as well.

_____

_____

_____

_____

_____

_____

PRACTICE THESE 10 MINDSET RULES:

1 Set big, bold, tremendous goals.

2 Be grateful for everything you have today, and everything you don't have yet.

3 Be 100% accountable for your life. It doesn't mean that everything is your fault, but taking 100% responsibility for it moves you forward with strength.

4 Be thankful – for everything that went well and for everything that didn't go well.

5 Act, speak, think, and perform from the perspective of your Goal Beyond The Goal®.

6 Replace every negative thought with positive thought.

7 Add enthusiasm, energy and certainty to everything in your life!

8 Disregard disempowering actions and language.

9 There are no problems, only opportunities.

10 Bring the data, not the drama!

week 3

MONDAY DAILY JOURNALING   DATE _____

MENTAL MINDSET FOR THE WEEK

Upgrade your goals. This book is teaching you how to have more control of
your outcomes. You've got this.

JOURNALING PROMPTS

O Pick an intentional word or phrase of the day that is directly related to your goals.
   What do you want?

_____

O Think about moving forward. What do you want to have in your A Circle? How will
   that support you? Today, practice putting more of *you* into your A Circle to move
   toward your goals.

_____
_____
_____
_____
_____
_____

O Think about what went well and what did not go well in the past. What strategies
   were you using in those situations? What was in your A Circle?

_____
_____
_____
_____
_____
_____

O How have your strategies evolved in the past three months? What are you more aware of? How have you been more accepting of yourself in your situation(s)?

_____

_____

_____

_____

_____

_____

O What goals have you achieved in the last three months? What strategies did you use to support those goals?

_____

_____

_____

_____

_____

_____

O What do you want to achieve in the next three months?

_____

_____

_____

_____

_____

_____

O What has been in your way of achieving your goals in the past? What is something that you don't want people to know about you? What limiting beliefs do you have about yourself, or your life, or your situation(s)?

_____

_____

_____

_____

_____

TUESDAY DAILY JOURNALING   DATE _____

JOURNALING PROMPTS

O Pick your intentional word or phrase of the day. Again, connect it directly to your goals.

_____

O How did yesterday's intentional word or phrase of the day support your goals? How can you support your goals more intentionally?

_____
_____
_____
_____
_____

O What is your goal beyond the goal? Where do you want to be 3 years down the road?

_____
_____
_____
_____
_____

O What is your goal for the next 3 months? What strategies do you use to support yourself in achieving your goals during these next 3 months?

_____
_____
_____
_____

O What do you do well? What do people say you do well? What are you good at in your sport and outside of your sport?

O Think of a situation where something went well. Go into that experience... and now step out of it. How were you doing that particular thing well? Was it something you saw? Something you felt? Something you said to yourself? Something you heard? Or a combination?

O This is your strategy for success. Can you use this more often? Where?

O Can you see how you can use this strategy to achieve your goals in the next 3 months? In the next 3 years? How could you have used it this past week?

O What inspired you today?

WEDNESDAY DAILY JOURNALING   DATE _____

JOURNALING PROMPTS

O Pick your intentional word or phrase of the day.

O How has the intentional word of the day changed how you live your life?

O Do you like to see your way through your skills/plays/sport? Or feel your way through, think your way through, talk your way through, or a combination?

O Think of a time when you were successful. What strategy were you using? What was in your A Circle?

O Can you practice using this strategy moving forward? In what past situations could you have used this strategy? With coaches? Teammates?

O Really dig down deep to think about what you do well. What gifts do you have that you can become more aware of? I want you to think about where things went really well in the past. How did you contribute to that?

O I am so proud of you. Get comfortable in your success. Know that you always have more to grow and do. BUT, get comfortable in it! We do not have to struggle to be more successful. Where in the past did you sabotage your success or yourself?

_____

_____

_____

_____

O Now, think about how you could have taken care of yourself better in those situations. Could you have gotten stronger without the injury? Could you have been better without struggling for the entire season?

_____

_____

_____

O Do you seek support from outside of yourself or inside of yourself? What works best for you? Do THAT more often. What ever works for you is great. Understanding what you need is what you can practice more.

_____

_____

_____

O Think about your situation. What are some great things about your situation (coaches...team...parents...club...school) that can support you to achieve your goals?

_____

_____

_____

O Outside of your sport —what do you love?

_____

_____

_____

_____

_____

THURSDAY DAILY JOURNALING   DATE _____

JOURNALING PROMPTS

O What is your intentional word of the day? Pick one that directly connects you to your gift!

_____

O Remember that you have a "present self "and a "goal self." Practice stepping out of your "present self" and stepping into your "goal self " more often. Add your ability to share your gift with the world more often. What do you do well and how do you do it well? How can you explore ways to do and be more of that??

_____

_____

_____

_____

O Do you have situations where your A Circle gets crowded with negative thoughts, or negative energy, or negative people? Are you having trouble kicking them out? If you are struggling with negative things in your A Circle, how can you replace them? Do you want to?

_____

_____

_____

_____

O For example, if you have fear/anxiety/worry in your A Circle, it is only there to help you pay attention, to think about what you want to be doing, or to remind yourself to focus on what you are doing physically. Practice thanking — yes thanking — that energy so you can use it to your advantage. Practice thanking *old* situations as well. What could you have done to support yourself better in the past?

_____

_____

_____

_____

O Think of some goals outside of your sport that you want to achieve. List them.

O Can you see how adding more of yourself to your goals outside of your sport adds more to your goals? How?

O We can only give away what we have inside ourselves. The great thing is that it will never take from us to support others when we have it for ourselves first. What do you see in others? If it is ugliness then love yourself more :)

I AM SO PROUD OF YOU!

FRIDAY DAILY JOURNALING   DATE _____

JOURNALING PROMPTS

O Pick your intentional word or phrase of the day. Think about your week. What can you focus on today that will support your entire week?

_____

O Can you think of situations this week where you were more in your own A Circle?

_____
_____
_____
_____

O How was that helpful for you?

_____
_____
_____
_____

O When you think about your A Circle, can you see how your ability to manage it can be helpful for your goals? What did you learn this week about how you are able to manage your A Circle?

_____
_____
_____
_____

O Think of situations in the past that did not go well. An injury? Maybe you broke down under pressure, or you were worried about what people were thinking of you. Write them down.

_____
_____
_____
_____

O Looking back, do you see that if you would have known these tools and strategies, they would have been helpful? Remember, you did the best you could with what you knew at the time. What strategies could you have used? What could you have had in your A Circle?

O This week, when you look back, name 3 reasons for your success.

O What do you do well? How do you do it well? Remember: nobody does your skills/ sport/game better than you —be confident in that.

O Step back and practice joy. Where do you have the most joy in your life? Do more of that.

SATURDAY DAILY JOURNALING   DATE _____

CELEBRATION DAY!

O Think of 5 situations where you were successful. Write them down.

_____

_____

_____

_____

_____

_____

O Think of 5 things that you accomplished this week. Write them down.

_____

_____

_____

_____

_____

_____

O Where did you build strength this week mentally? Physically?

_____

_____

_____

_____

_____

O What did you learn from this week that can support you to achieve your goals?

_____

_____

_____

_____

_____

O What went well? What didn't go well? And what can you learn from both?

O Remember that you are not equal to the result. When you accomplish a goal, it is fantastic —*but you are not equal to it.* Learn from it so you can use that experience and same strategy to build success. Where this week can you use this?

O Also, you are not equal to the mistake, or what did not go well. Separate yourself from those situations so that you can also learn from them. Can you think of any situation this week where you can practice this? Are you hard on yourself? Do you have high expectations of yourself? That's okay, but neither of those things belong in your A Circle when you are doing your sport. Did you have situations this week where this got in your way?

SUNDAY! DAILY JOURNALING   DATE _____

DREAM DAY!

○ Give yourself permission to dream. We need to practice dreaming. It's not a bad thing to desire, or to want things in your life! Putting your best self into your life, sharing your gift to the world, being more of you, is your responsibility and your job. Dreaming only inspires more of you in that way. As you practice putting more of you into your life, you can share that with others; that is inspiring. Where this week were you more of you?

_____

_____

_____

_____

_____

○ Regarding your answer above, were people receptive to it or a little bit threatened?

_____

_____

_____

Remember this: I can only see in you what I have in myself. So, if I don't see you in all your brightness, it's not because something is wrong with *you*. It is *my* lack that is the issue. Do not let someone else's inability to see your light dim it. Practice being your light. Practice seeing other's light as well.

_____

_____

_____

_____

_____

_____

_____

_____

PRACTICE THESE 10 MINDSET RULES:

1 Set big, bold, tremendous goals.

2 Be grateful for everything you have today, and everything you don't have yet.

3 Be 100% accountable for your life. It doesn't mean that everything is your fault, but taking 100% responsibility for it moves you forward with strength.

4 Be thankful – for everything that went well and for everything that didn't go well.

5 Act, speak, think, and perform from the perspective of your Goal Beyond The Goal®.

6 Replace every negative thought with positive thought.

7 Add enthusiasm, energy and certainty to everything in your life!

8 Disregard disempowering actions and language.

9 There are no problems, only opportunities.

10 Bring the data, not the drama!

week 4
MONDAY DAILY JOURNALING DATE _____

MENTAL MINDSET FOR THE WEEK

Remember that once you set a goal, it is seeking you as much as you are seeking it!
Pay attention to how it is coming to you!

JOURNALING PROMPTS

O Pick an intentional word or phrase of the day that is directly related to your goals.
What do you want?

_____

O Think about moving forward. What do you want to have in your A Circle? How will
that support you? Today, practice putting more of *you* into your A Circle to move
toward your goals.

_____
_____
_____
_____
_____
_____
_____

O Think about what went well and what did not go well in the past. What strategies
were you using in those situations? What was in your A Circle?

_____
_____
_____
_____
_____
_____

O How have your strategies evolved in the past three months? What are you more aware of? How have you been more accepting of yourself in your situation(s)?

O What goals have you achieved in the last three months? What strategies did you use to support those goals?

O What do you want to achieve in the next three months?

O What has been in your way of achieving your goals in the past? What is something that you don't want people to know about you? What limiting beliefs do you have about yourself, or your life, or your situation(s)?

TUESDAY DAILY JOURNALING   DATE _____

JOURNALING PROMPTS

O Pick your intentional word or phrase of the day. Again, connect it directly to your goals.

_____

O How did yesterday's intentional word or phrase of the day support your goals? How can you support your goals more intentionally?

_____
_____
_____
_____
_____

O What is your goal beyond the goal? Where do you want to be 3 years down the road?

_____
_____
_____
_____
_____

O What is your goal for the next 3 months? What strategies do you use to support yourself in achieving your goals during these next 3 months?

_____
_____
_____
_____

MENTAL STRENGTH COACHING JOURNAL   221

O   What do you do well? What do people say you do well? What are you good at in
    your sport and outside of your sport?

O   Think of a situation where something went well. Go into that experience... and
    now step out of it. How were you doing that particular thing well? Was it some-
    thing you saw? Something you felt? Something you said to yourself? Something
    you heard? Or a combination?

O   This is your strategy for success. Can you use this more often? Where?

O   Can you see how you can use this strategy to achieve your goals in the next 3
    months? In the next 3 years? How could you have used it this past week?

O   What inspired you today?

WEDNESDAY DAILY JOURNALING   DATE _____

JOURNALING PROMPTS

O Pick your intentional word or phrase of the day.

_____

O How has the intentional word of the day changed how you live your life?

_____

_____

O Do you like to see your way through your skills/plays/sport? Or feel your way
   through, think your way through, talk your way through, or a combination?

_____

_____

_____

O Think of a time when you were successful. What strategy were you using? What
   was in your A Circle?

_____

_____

_____

O Can you practice using this strategy moving forward? In what past situations could
   you have used this strategy? With coaches? Teammates?

_____

_____

_____

O Really dig down deep to think about what you do well. What gifts do you have that
   you can become more aware of? I want you to think about where things went really
   well in the past. How did you contribute to that?

_____

_____

_____

O I am so proud of you. Get comfortable in your success. Know that you always have more to grow and do. BUT, get comfortable in it! We do not have to struggle to be more successful. Where in the past did you sabotage your success or yourself?

_____

_____

_____

_____

O Now, think about how you could have taken care of yourself better in those situations. Could you have gotten stronger without the injury? Could you have been better without struggling for the entire season?

_____

_____

_____

O Do you seek support from outside of yourself or inside of yourself? What works best for you? Do THAT more often. What ever works for you is great. Understanding what you need is what you can practice more.

_____

_____

_____

O Think about your situation. What are some great things about your situation (coaches...team...parents...club...school) that can support you to achieve your goals?

_____

_____

_____

O Outside of your sport —what do you love?

_____

_____

_____

_____

_____

THURSDAY DAILY JOURNALING   DATE _____

JOURNALING PROMPTS

O What is your intentional word of the day? Pick one that directly connects you to your gift!

_____

O Remember that you have a "present self "and a "goal self." Practice stepping out of your "present self" and stepping into your "goal self " more often. Add your ability to share your gift with the world more often. What do you do well and how do you do it well? How can you explore ways to do and be more of that??

_____

_____

_____

_____

O Do you have situations where your A Circle gets crowded with negative thoughts, or negative energy, or negative people? Are you having trouble kicking them out? If you are struggling with negative things in your A Circle, how can you replace them? Do you want to?

_____

_____

_____

_____

O For example, if you have fear/anxiety/worry in your A Circle, it is only there to help you pay attention, to think about what you want to be doing, or to remind yourself to focus on what you are doing physically. Practice thanking — yes thanking — that energy so you can use it to your advantage. Practice thanking *old* situations as well. What could you have done to support yourself better in the past?

_____

_____

_____

MENTAL STRENGTH COACHING JOURNAL   225

O Think of some goals outside of your sport that you want to achieve. List them.

O Can you see how adding more of yourself to your goals outside of your sport adds more to your goals? How?

O We can only give away what we have inside ourselves. The great thing is that it will never take from us to support others when we have it for ourselves first. What do you see in others? If it is ugliness then love yourself more :)

I AM SO PROUD OF YOU!

FRIDAY DAILY JOURNALING   DATE _____

JOURNALING PROMPTS

O Pick your intentional word or phrase of the day. Think about your week. What can you focus on today that will support your entire week?

_____

O Can you think of situations this week where you were more in your own A Circle?

_____
_____
_____
_____

O How was that helpful for you?

_____
_____
_____
_____

O When you think about your A Circle, can you see how your ability to manage it can be helpful for your goals? What did you learn this week about how you are able to manage your A Circle?

_____
_____
_____
_____

O Think of situations in the past that did not go well. An injury? Maybe you broke down under pressure, or you were worried about what people were thinking of you. Write them down.

_____
_____
_____
_____

MENTAL STRENGTH COACHING JOURNAL   227

O Looking back, do you see that if you would have known these tools and strategies, they would have been helpful? Remember, you did the best you could with what you knew at the time. What strategies could you have used? What could you have had in your A Circle?

O This week, when you look back, name 3 reasons for your success.

O What do you do well? How do you do it well? Remember: nobody does your skills/ sport/game better than you —be confident in that.

O Step back and practice joy. Where do you have the most joy in your life? Do more of that.

SATURDAY DAILY JOURNALING   DATE _____

CELEBRATION DAY!

○ Think of 5 situations where you were successful. Write them down.

_____

_____

_____

_____

_____

_____

○ Think of 5 things that you accomplished this week. Write them down.

_____

_____

_____

_____

_____

_____

○ Where did you build strength this week mentally? Physically?

_____

_____

_____

_____

_____

_____

○ What did you learn from this week that can support you to achieve your goals?

_____

_____

_____

_____

_____

_____

MENTAL STRENGTH COACHING JOURNAL   229

O What went well? What didn't go well? And what can you learn from both?

O Remember that you are not equal to the result. When you accomplish a goal, it is fantastic —*but you are not equal to it.* Learn from it so you can use that experience and same strategy to build success. Where this week can you use this?

O Also, you are not equal to the mistake, or what did not go well. Separate yourself from those situations so that you can also learn from them. Can you think of any situation this week where you can practice this? Are you hard on yourself? Do you have high expectations of yourself? That's okay, but neither of those things belong in your A Circle when you are doing your sport. Did you have situations this week where this got in your way?

SUNDAY! DAILY JOURNALING   DATE _____

DREAM DAY!

O Give yourself permission to dream. We need to practice dreaming. It's not a bad
thing to desire, or to want things in your life! Putting your best self into your life,
sharing your gift to the world, being more of you, is your responsibility and your
job. Dreaming only inspires more of you in that way. As you practice putting more
of you into your life, you can share that with others; that is inspiring. Where this
week were you more of you?

_____

_____

_____

_____

_____

O Regarding your answer above, were people receptive to it or a little bit threatened?

_____

_____

_____

Remember this: I can only see in you what I have in myself. So, if I
don't see you in all your brightness, it's not because something is
wrong with *you*. It is *my* lack that is the issue. Do not let someone
else's inability to see your light dim it. Practice being your light.
Practice seeing other's light as well.

_____

_____

_____

_____

_____

_____

PRACTICE THESE 10 MINDSET RULES:

1 Set big, bold, tremendous goals.

2 Be grateful for everything you have today, and everything you don't have yet.

3 Be 100% accountable for your life. It doesn't mean that everything is your fault, but taking 100% responsibility for it moves you forward with strength.

4 Be thankful – for everything that went well and for everything that didn't go well.

5 Act, speak, think, and perform from the perspective of your Goal Beyond The Goal®.

6 Replace every negative thought with positive thought.

7 Add enthusiasm, energy and certainty to everything in your life!

8 Disregard disempowering actions and language.

9 There are no problems, only opportunities.

10 Bring the data, not the drama!

week 5

MONDAY DAILY JOURNALING   DATE _____

MENTAL MINDSET FOR THE WEEK

Yay! You made it! See you on Book 3! I'm so proud of you!

JOURNALING PROMPTS

O Pick an intentional word or phrase of the day that is directly related to your goals. What do you want?

_____

O Think about moving forward. What do you want to have in your A Circle? How will that support you? Today, practice putting more of *you* into your A Circle to move toward your goals.

_____
_____
_____
_____
_____
_____

O Think about what went well and what did not go well in the past. What strategies were you using in those situations? What was in your A Circle?

_____
_____
_____
_____
_____
_____

MENTAL STRENGTH COACHING JOURNAL   233

O How have your strategies evolved in the past three months? What are you more aware of? How have you been more accepting of yourself in your situation(s)?

O What goals have you achieved in the last three months? What strategies did you use to support those goals?

O What do you want to achieve in the next three months?

O What has been in your way of achieving your goals in the past? What is something that you don't want people to know about you? What limiting beliefs do you have about yourself, or your life, or your situation(s)?

TUESDAY DAILY JOURNALING   DATE _____

JOURNALING PROMPTS

O Pick your intentional word or phrase of the day. Again, connect it directly to your goals.

_____

O How did yesterday's intentional word or phrase of the day support your goals? How can you support your goals more intentionally?

_____
_____
_____
_____
_____

O What is your goal beyond the goal? Where do you want to be 3 years down the road?

_____
_____
_____
_____
_____

O What is your goal for the next 3 months? What strategies do you use to support yourself in achieving your goals during these next 3 months?

_____
_____
_____

O What do you do well? What do people say you do well? What are you good at in your sport and outside of your sport?

_____

_____

_____

_____

O Think of a situation where something went well. Go into that experience... and now step out of it. How were you doing that particular thing well? Was it something you saw? Something you felt? Something you said to yourself? Something you heard? Or a combination?

_____

_____

_____

_____

O This is your strategy for success. Can you use this more often? Where?

_____

_____

_____

_____

O Can you see how you can use this strategy to achieve your goals in the next 3 months? In the next 3 years? How could you have used it this past week?

_____

_____

_____

_____

O What inspired you today?

_____

_____

_____

_____

WEDNESDAY DAILY JOURNALING   DATE _____

JOURNALING PROMPTS

O Pick your intentional word or phrase of the day.

_____

O How has the intentional word of the day changed how you live your life?

_____
_____

O Do you like to see your way through your skills/plays/sport? Or feel your way through, think your way through, talk your way through, or a combination?

_____
_____
_____

O Think of a time when you were successful. What strategy were you using? What was in your A Circle?

_____
_____
_____

O Can you practice using this strategy moving forward? In what past situations could you have used this strategy? With coaches? Teammates?

_____
_____
_____

O Really dig down deep to think about what you do well. What gifts do you have that you can become more aware of? I want you to think about where things went really well in the past. How did you contribute to that?

_____
_____
_____

○ I am so proud of you. Get comfortable in your success. Know that you always have more to grow and do. BUT, get comfortable in it! We do not have to struggle to be more successful. Where in the past did you sabotage your success or yourself?

○ Now, think about how you could have taken care of yourself better in those situations. Could you have gotten stronger without the injury? Could you have been better without struggling for the entire season?

○ Do you seek support from outside of yourself or inside of yourself? What works best for you? Do THAT more often. What ever works for you is great. Understanding what you need is what you can practice more.

○ Think about your situation. What are some great things about your situation (coaches...team...parents...club...school) that can support you to achieve your goals?

○ Outside of your sport —what do you love?

THURSDAY DAILY JOURNALING   DATE _____

JOURNALING PROMPTS

O What is your intentional word of the day? Pick one that directly connects you to your gift!

_____

O Remember that you have a "present self "and a "goal self." Practice stepping out of your "present self" and stepping into your "goal self " more often. Add your ability to share your gift with the world more often. What do you do well and how do you do it well? How can you explore ways to do and be more of that??

_____

_____

_____

O Do you have situations where your A Circle gets crowded with negative thoughts, or negative energy, or negative people? Are you having trouble kicking them out? If you are struggling with negative things in your A Circle, how can you replace them? Do you want to?

_____

_____

_____

O For example, if you have fear/anxiety/worry in your A Circle, it is only there to help you pay attention, to think about what you want to be doing, or to remind yourself to focus on what you are doing physically. Practice thanking — yes thanking — that energy so you can use it to your advantage. Practice thanking *old* situations as well. What could you have done to support yourself better in the past?

_____

_____

_____

O Think of some goals outside of your sport that you want to achieve. List them.

O Can you see how adding more of yourself to your goals outside of your sport adds more to your goals? How?

O We can only give away what we have inside ourselves. The great thing is that it will never take from us to support others when we have it for ourselves first. What do you see in others? If it is ugliness then love yourself more :)

I AM SO PROUD OF YOU!

FRIDAY DAILY JOURNALING   DATE _____

JOURNALING PROMPTS

O Pick your intentional word or phrase of the day. Think about your week. What can you focus on today that will support your entire week?

_____

O Can you think of situations this week where you were more in your own A Circle?

_____
_____
_____
_____

O How was that helpful for you?

_____
_____
_____
_____

O When you think about your A Circle, can you see how your ability to manage it can be helpful for your goals? What did you learn this week about how you are able to manage your A Circle?

_____
_____
_____
_____

O Think of situations in the past that did not go well. An injury? Maybe you broke down under pressure, or you were worried about what people were thinking of you. Write them down.

_____
_____
_____
_____

O Looking back, do you see that if you would have known these tools and strategies, they would have been helpful? Remember, you did the best you could with what you knew at the time. What strategies could you have used? What could you have had in your A Circle?

O This week, when you look back, name 3 reasons for your success.

O What do you do well? How do you do it well? Remember: nobody does your skills/ sport/game better than you —be confident in that.

O Step back and practice joy. Where do you have the most joy in your life? Do more of that.

SATURDAY DAILY JOURNALING — DATE _____

CELEBRATION DAY!

O Think of 5 situations where you were successful. Write them down.

_____
_____
_____
_____
_____
_____

O Think of 5 things that you accomplished this week. Write them down.

_____
_____
_____
_____
_____
_____

O Where did you build strength this week mentally? Physically?

_____
_____
_____
_____
_____
_____

O What did you learn from this week that can support you to achieve your goals?

_____
_____
_____
_____
_____
_____

- What went well? What didn't go well? And what can you learn from both?

- Remember that you are not equal to the result. When you accomplish a goal, it is fantastic —*but you are not equal to it*. Learn from it so you can use that experience and same strategy to build success. Where this week can you use this?

- Also, you are not equal to the mistake, or what did not go well. Separate yourself from those situations so that you can also learn from them. Can you think of any situation this week where you can practice this? Are you hard on yourself? Do you have high expectations of yourself? That's okay, but neither of those things belong in your A Circle when you are doing your sport. Did you have situations this week where this got in your way?

SUNDAY! DAILY JOURNALING   DATE _____

DREAM DAY!

O Give yourself permission to dream. We need to practice dreaming. It's not a bad thing to desire, or to want things in your life! Putting your best self into your life, sharing your gift to the world, being more of you, is your responsibility and your job. Dreaming only inspires more of you in that way. As you practice putting more of you into your life, you can share that with others; that is inspiring. Where this week were you more of you?

_____

_____

_____

_____

_____

O Regarding your answer above, were people receptive to it or a little bit threatened?

_____

_____

_____

Remember this: I can only see in you what I have in myself. So, if I don't see you in all your brightness, it's not because something is wrong with *you*. It is *my* lack that is the issue. Do not let someone else's inability to see your light dim it. Practice being your light. Practice seeing other's light as well.

_____

_____

_____

_____

_____

_____

PRACTICE THESE 10 MINDSET RULES:

1 Set big, bold, tremendous goals.

2 Be grateful for everything you have today, and everything you don't have yet.

3 Be 100% accountable for your life. It doesn't mean that everything is your fault, but taking 100% responsibility for it moves you forward with strength.

4 Be thankful – for everything that went well and for everything that didn't go well.

5 Act, speak, think, and perform from the perspective of your Goal Beyond The Goal®.

6 Replace every negative thought with positive thought.

7 Add enthusiasm, energy and certainty to everything in your life!

8 Disregard disempowering actions and language.

9 There are no problems, only opportunities.

10 Bring the data, not the drama!

246 MENTAL STRENGTH COACHING JOURNAL

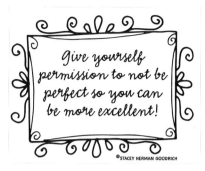
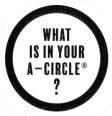
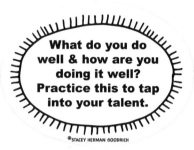
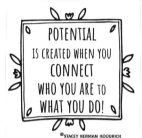
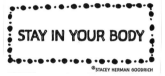
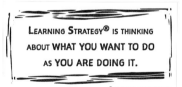
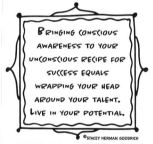
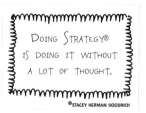
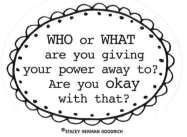